Cancer Free!

HOW TO RECEIVE HEALING FROM GOD, ESPECIALLY IF YOU DON'T DESERVE IT.

PHILIP LANDRY

Paperback ISBN: 978-0-578-83636-2
Ebook ISBN: 978-0-578-83491-7

The following translations and versions are referred to: NIV (New International Version), NKJV (New King James Version), NASB (New American Standard Bible), CJB (Complete Jewish Bible), ESV (English Standard Version), MSG (The Message Bible) and I think the KJV (King James Version - public domain).

Dedication

I'd like to dedicate this book to my loving Lord and Savior, Jesus Christ, who loved me and loves me in spite of myself. And to my wife, Penny, who loved me with her love throughout this journey and for most of my life. To me, you are so beautiful and radiant and kind and... (I could go on but I think you'd prefer I say this in person). Finally, to my children. First, for letting me love them. It is such a blessing to love others and I am whole in my soul when I can love you, however imperfect this love is for each of you. Secondly, for loving me in return in your own unique way. I cannot imagine life without any of you.

Acknowledgments

There are so many people to acknowledge. My apologies if I missed anyone. My parents, for loving me in spite of the challenges I gave them. My friends Bob and Dareda Mueller, for praying for me and loving me when I could not return this love. For those who cared for me in the hospital where I stayed, who were either encouraging, funny, or helpful in some way. For those who came to visit in my first few days (I don't remember anyone). For Pastor Aaron, as a young pastor, you were gracious, kind, and pointed to Jesus. And for your own mentor who told you to "let me have what I was saying". For that, I will be forever grateful as you did not upset my wife with death counseling. For Pastor Joseph Prince, for your encouraging word and encouraging words. It is so easy to read the good that God is from your published writings and your spoken teachings. My distant cousin, Matt Landry, for encouraging me on the details for publishing and with a timeline to get the book published (which I didn't hit but came close to doing). I trust this book will be an encouragement to others as your books are to your own audience. To my editor, N. Amma Twum-Baah, who helped me tell the story in addition to helping me to pull it together from a flow standpoint. And to Brent Spears, for his help in pulling together a beautiful Cover design and formatting that makes it easy on the eyes.

Because I didn't get a chance to ask everyone who is in the book for their permission to use their name, I changed all of the names except, of course, for myself, my wife, my children and their spouses. If we catch up and you give me your okay, I'll update the electronic versions of the book.

CONTENTS

1. The Beginning of My End 1

2. Finding Cancer 7

3. At Death's Door 19

4. My Bargaining Nature Kicks In 25

5. Fallen from Grace 30

6. Healing Isn't Surviving! 36

7. Who You Lookin' at Anyway? 46

8. The Pressure Is on Him, Not You 52

9. The Father's Love for You 57

10. Become Jesus Conscious 65

11. What Do You "Do" To Receive Healing? 70

12. His Purpose in His Life for You 88

13. Faith Hears What God Says 101

14. The End of My Beginning. 110

1.

THE BEGINNING OF MY END

In 2014, I was healed of the most aggressive form of stage-four non-Hodgkin's lymphoma. This book tells the story of how I was healed of what was a "triple hit lymphoma" diagnosis. I hope my story will encourage everyone who reads it and will give you assurance that God loves you, God wants you healed, and God hates death and sickness and He loves life with you. I'll be quoting scripture, but I'm not looking to make anyone a bible scholar, nor do you have to be a scholar to be healed. You must simply trust that God has provided everything you need for your well-being through His Son, the Messiah, Jesus the Christ. I am a living testament to what is possible with God. I have all the tests I went through and even some videos of the PET scans I underwent, as proof that God is my healer.

All of the names in this story have been changed because some requested that I do so; others, I simply didn't have time to get their permission. However, this story is real. Everything happened exactly as I have shared it. I'm giving you my hindsight as I look back on the steps my wife and I took, why we took those steps and did what we did, and what impact all of it had on my healing. I'm going to lay out the biggest takeaway from this book right up front. I need you to believe that God is in love with you. He loves you so much that He wants you healed, or He wants your loved one healed. His love for you was demonstrated on the cross when He gave His only begotten Son so that you might live. Believe in Jesus! Believe in His love for you. I'm going to focus on how you receive from God. Nothing I share is difficult. He has the hard part. I simply want you to know and believe in the love that He has for you.

So, who am I? I'm the oldest of six children and perhaps the most rebellious of my siblings. Earlier in my marriage and family life, I was also the most self-righteous about my beliefs after I came to have a living relationship with God. I believed that my good works and the fact that I "believed" put me in good stead with God. That because I did good, I deserved to be treated accordingly. I also used to believe that those who don't believe in God's word were misguided folks who didn't know the error of their ways. Behind this self-righteousness was a fear that took on many masks. Sometimes, this fear took on the mask of anger, sometimes ridicule, sometimes smugness. I'm a fun-loving human being, but I was also a stern father. The majority of the time, I knew how to keep myself in check, but my frustration would rise when things were not going my way, and that gave rise to anger with my wife and sometimes with my children.

Being the oldest, I easily took on most responsibilities with great confidence. People sometimes mistook my confidence for arrogance. This confidence served me well as my sales career flourished. My wife and I went on many sales club trips together. We enjoyed many trips to Hawaii, a staple for many sales organizations, and enjoyed free travel to Puerto Rico, Mexico (Acapulco and Cancun), further places like Tahiti/Bora Bora, and the island of Madeira (part of Portugal off the coast of Africa). One year, I was fortunate enough to be number one worldwide in sales for a multi-billion-dollar software company, and in addition to going on the club trip to Cancun, Mexico, we decided to take a month off and trek throughout Europe with our teenage daughters along for the ride. Life was good and I was enjoying the blessings of God.

When I first met my wife, I had just graduated from the University of Chicago and was working in the downtown area of Chicago. To keep myself grounded, I meditated in a Buddhist temple on the near north side twice a week. It was an exercise I eagerly undertook to help keep me centered. However, I would easily fall asleep in meditation practice. When this happened, I was rewarded with a light whack on the back of my head with a small bamboo stick by my loving Zen master. In Zen Buddhism, they use riddles to describe reaching a state of contentment or a state of "no-striving" or ease. An example of this was understanding what "the sound of one hand clapping" was. I believe I had reached this state in my spirit. This resting without striving was what I wanted in my life.

I lived near Lincoln Park on the north side of Chicago, so I would often go there on weekends simply to walk and enjoy the serenity of the city park. I loved Chicago. There was so much going on. Busy-ness everywhere. I found this relaxing because I find peace in chaotic situations. My father had always wanted me to be a doctor or a lawyer and if I had chosen the medical profession, I would have enjoyed being an emergency room doctor because when all hell breaks loose, it gives me peace inside. I must focus and zero in on what's important and block out what's unnecessary to accomplish the task at hand. This act of focusing on what's important gives me a sense of peace. I think I received this nature from my earthly father and it probably did him well going through the chaos of both World War II and later the Korean War.

One Saturday afternoon, sitting on a park bench in Lincoln Park, I began to think of how wonderful it would be to share my life with another person. Someone who understood 'the sound of one-hand clapping', I thought. It was like I was sharing this thought with some universal God who understood what I needed because, the very next week, I met the woman of my dreams who would later become my wife. I met Penny for the first time on a bus heading into downtown Chicago. It was as if God had heard and answered my thoughts. While we took that bus route every day for the next year, we never again met on that bus route heading into Chicago. Penny became my life partner almost from the moment we first met.

We are different. Extremely different. Like night and day. Opposites to be exact. I can be demanding. She is easy going. I can't dance. She loves to express herself with dance in a delicate way, almost like she is a flower blooming under the sun. She has rarely said an ugly word about anyone since we met. I have no problem telling people what I think to their face, let alone behind their backs. Sometimes, that has gotten me into trouble. Most times, it's gotten me into trouble with my love, my Penny. Her demands are always indirect. For example, after we started getting serious in our courtship, she told me that she would never marry someone who didn't know Jesus Christ. Her way wasn't to force or demand that I do anything. But I had no interest in this God who seemed to me, to be contradictory and judgmental, and only wanted me to perform for Him, but, for the sake of our relationship, I went along with it just so I could be with her. I was so drawn to her that when I looked at her, my heart would sometimes buckle in weakness over this desire to be with her.

During our courtship, I set out to prove that this "bible" was just a bunch of baloney. Man-made stuff. But the more I studied it, the more I realized that I didn't know what I was talking about. I could see how perfect this word of God was. The way it is written, the patterns in that word, when things were spoken, and when they weren't. As I saw that this word of God could be true, I began to trust it more. God was good and only wanted good for my life. He knew what was best for me and His way was gentle with me.

I'm not God. I stumble. When people come to the word of

God, they come to it with their baggage, their strengths, and their abilities. And even though these abilities are from God, we own them. We call them good qualities, and sometimes we wish people had the same innate qualities that we were given by God. "*If only people were like me, the world would be a better place,*" I would think. I had no trouble believing God's word. But sometimes I had great trouble with people who struggled with believing God's word. This surfaced with my wife and later with my three girls. For example, God was blessing me with sales, but *I* made the sales. *I* believed for the sales. *I* got it done. I, I, I. This line of thinking happens to everyone. For example, my wife is extraordinarily kind. This is a natural ability for her, so she naturally thinks that everyone should be kind like her. People must be godly because they're kind. Back and forth this reasoning went, sometimes surfacing in normal conversations with her, other times in high pitched arguments.

It's dangerous to think that if only people were like us, the world would be a better place. I think that we all have some degree of self-righteousness about abilities that are unique to us. Qualities we have that are good. Why can't others just be like me? However, when you think like this, it becomes more difficult to understand others. My wife and I had many challenges together because of my thinking. She had her strengths and I had mine and they never got along very well. We were so different. We'd argue and yell with me mostly doing the yelling. And we'd disagree on what to do almost all the time. I never thought through why I was attracted to someone so different from me, but I believe God wanted to show me how much He loved me by giving me someone so different to love. God is good like that.

I am an imperfect man who wants you to know that I was healed of stage-four Non-Hodgkin's lymphoma by a perfect man. His name is Jesus Christ. He is the Messiah and my Messiah. I want to point you to Him and not to me. But I want you to understand the struggles I had and why I was still healed despite those struggles.

He loved me and He loves me. I want you to believe that He loves you too. Not because you deserve to be loved because of something you do or did for Him. Not because you're nice in your own eyes. The more I realized I was loved by God, the easier it became for me to love someone so different from me, my Penny. Just as it's physically healing to be in her arms, it is physically healing to be in the arms of my Savior, to know the Messiah who loves me. This is my story of the love of my Messiah *for me*.

2.

FINDING CANCER

I remember lying in a hospital bed, propped up with pillows and staring down at my two very swollen legs, wondering, "*How did it come to this? How in the world did I get here?*" My legs looked the size of small tree trunks and my voice had a gravelly tone to it when I spoke. It was as if I now had the voice of Clint Eastwood. I even began to imagine Clint and I collaborating on the story of how I got there in that hospital bed. For the most part, I floated in and out of consciousness because I was tired. I tend to sleep a lot when I'm tired. I've never had any difficulty falling asleep within seconds of hitting the pillow.

By now I'd been in the hospital for a few days. I couldn't tell exactly how long, but people kept coming in and out of the hospital room. Doctors, nurses, and people who wanted to see me. All while I lay there trying to understand the path that had gotten me there. It was a futile exercise. Medicines were flowing into my body and the constant beep, beep, beep of medical instruments created an intense musical cacophony contributing to the anxiety in the room. I sensed that things had taken a scary turn. I couldn't pin it down, but I realized that I might not be here much longer. I occasionally heard someone in another room moaning loudly in pain. I lay quiet, facing my feet and wondering to myself, "*how on earth did I get here?*"

A few months earlier, Penny and I had gone out to dinner to try out the newest restaurant in our neighborhood. We were a few bites into the main course when I started experiencing a dull pain in my stomach area. I tried not to think too much of it even though the pain was strong enough to get my attention. We made it through dinner and got back home, and that's when the pain intensified. Advil provided only temporary relief from the pain.

Over the several days that followed, I continued to work in my home office, making business calls, taking a few Advil pain killers, and getting a few hours of sleep each night. It was a pattern that I failed to recognize. Cancer doesn't just show up at your doorstep one day to dance with you. A month earlier, I had felt weak, so weak that I bought a shower chair at Walmart so I could sit in the shower. It was simply too hard to stand. All I could do was sit in the shower. I didn't think anything of it. Perhaps it was just a phase I was going through. *It would soon pass*, I thought. The dull stomach aches continued with more frequency and the pains became sharper. I'm sure eating liquid Advil like candy wasn't good for my stomach either, but it provided temporary relief to the relentless onslaught of pain.

But the more I took pain relievers, the more pain I experienced. Each night, I had less sleep than I had the night before. It had gotten so bad that I began to pray aloud while pacing back and forth in my bedroom. My pacing was quiet but deliberate because I didn't want to wake up my wife. Standing up seemed to provide temporary relief while pacing back and forth from the bed to the chair and back to the bed again. With each step, the pain gave me a renewed sense of urgency. *This has gotta stop*, I thought.

Five days after that meal at the restaurant, I woke up at 3 a.m. with stabbing pains in my stomach. I couldn't take it anymore, so

I decided to leave our bedroom and head into the hallway to call a friend.

Johnny was blind due to a freak firecracker accident and had been living without sight for the past ten to twelve years. For him, it was difficult to track when it was daytime or nighttime, so I knew Johnny would be up. "Hi Johnny, I greeted him when he answered the phone, "how are you?" Johnny responded to my greeting with an enthusiastic, "Fantastic Phil! 'As He is, so are we in this world,'[1]" This was one of Johnny's favorite phrases with which he loved to greet almost everyone. I never felt sorry for Johnny and he didn't want my pity either.

I was in too much pain for small talk, so I spoke quickly. "Johnny, I don't know what it is, but I'm in excruciating pain in my stomach area right now and I need someone ... I need you to pray for me."

Johnny responded with his gentle focused demeanor. This was an opportunity for him to invoke the power of God. He prayed for me by calling out God's good graces over me.

After his brief prayer, Johnny did what so many other people do as their first inclination - he tried to diagnose my problem. Because we all know that if there's a problem, we need to understand why it happened, right? That's the way the world works. "What have you been doing lately?" Johnny asked me. "What do you mean Johnny?" I quickly replied. I wanted to get off the phone because I knew what was coming next. "Well, what's happening in your life to *cause* this?" Johnny persisted. "I don't know Johnny," I said, brushing him off. Why focus on the problem, I thought.

Johnny was looking for dirt and I wasn't going to give him any, so I simply and politely said to him, "I'm fine, Johnny. Thanks for praying for me. I've got to go and get some rest now." Letting go of the issue, Johnny replied, "God bless you brother. You have

---

[1] 1 John 4:17 (NKJV) *Love has been perfected among us in this: that we may have boldness in the day of judgment; because as He is, so are we in this world.*

been healed by the stripes of Jesus Christ." I replied, "Amen to that Johnny. I'll talk to you later. Love you, my friend," and hung up the phone and sat in my reclining chair by the bed and tried to fall asleep.

The chair allowed me to stretch out and lay back, leaving me slightly propped up. This position provided me with much-needed relief and allowed me to doze off within minutes. But minutes later, I was hit by another wave of pain, this one more severe than the last. I pushed myself up and out of the chair and walked over and knelt beside our bed to pray. Quietly I said, "God, you have healed me by the stripes of Jesus Christ. Pain, I command you, leave my body, in Jesus' name I pray, Amen!" Still, the pain persisted. Why? What was wrong? It seemed stronger than ever, and after pacing the floor and praying, I gave up. I gently nudged Penny awake and told her we had to go to the hospital. I couldn't control this pain and it was too much for me to bear at that point.

We both got dressed and rushed to the closest emergency room ten minutes away. When we got there, I filled out the paperwork at the front desk. The pain coursing through my body was now urgent. "*I don't need this paperwork,*" I thought. Penny and I sat in the waiting room for a few minutes after filling out the paperwork and then I was ushered into a place surrounded by drapes. You could hear every pain from behind every curtain as if they were all singing out of tune. Waves of stomach pain flooded my body again and I stood and paced the floor. "Where is the doctor? Why is it taking them so long to see me?" I scowled at my wife. Poor Penny was closest to me and so I took out this anger on her. In response, she did what she has always done, she confessed God's word as if it were true. "Phil, by Jesus Christ's stripes, you are healed." It was true, but when you're in pain, you're not in a state to focus on that truth.

After what seemed like an eternity, but had only been about thirty to forty minutes, someone came by. I explained to the doctor what was going on. Stomach pains. For the past four to five days, each day, the pain had gotten worse than the day before. I explained to the doctor that the last thing I remembered was going to a restaurant and having food and cheap wine. So, maybe it was food poisoning.

"It hurts, Doctor, can you do anything about it now?" I pleaded with her. "Well, we need to take a more careful look at this," she replied. "We'll prep you for a CAT Scan and then decide what course of action to take." Unfortunately, she wasn't going to be rushed into a decision.

A few minutes went by before a male nurse came in. He seemed upset; not with me, but at something in his life. He gave me a shot, sticking me with force. In his mind, it seemed I wasn't there. I think he was sticking it to whomever he was mad at. *This guy shouldn't be a nurse*, I thought. Minutes after he left, my arm still smarted from his attack. Then someone came in and gave me a special drink for the CAT Scan and informed me that they would scan me in about thirty minutes. Pain was my companion now, sometimes throbbing, sometimes sharp. Time wasn't happening fast enough.

The next morning, after a CAT scan, a colonoscopy, and an EGD (it's a scope that goes down your throat to look at the stomach area), I was back in the recovery room. Everything went well, I was told. They had detected a few swollen lymph nodes on the CAT scan, but it was nothing to be concerned about. They also said that I may have to be treated for an ulcer but, besides that, everything was fine. I needed the floor doctor to approve my discharge, so they asked me to wait for his approval before I could go home. He would be making his rounds shortly, they told me. Hearing this, I tried to be on my best behavior. I wanted, no, I needed to get out of there. There is something about hospitals that makes me feel like I'm in the wrong place.

I pushed to put my game face on, despite feeling groggy from the lingering effects of the anesthesia. When the doctor came into the room, I said the most enthusiastic "hi" I could muster. "How do you feel?" the doctor asked me. "Great", I responded, "when can I leave?" Not what was wrong with me and not what did I have, but "when can I leave?" The doctor seemed puzzled by this response, but only for a moment. He brushed aside my comment and went into his prepared speech. "We did a colonoscopy and an EGD and we're going to recommend you see a gastroenterologist." I smiled weakly, trying to show some alertness. He recommended a gastroenterologist for me, signed the chart and I was on my way out of that place.

Penny and I eventually met the gastroenterologist who proceeded to treat me for an ulcer I did not have. Because of the continual pain and because of the impact on my stomach lining, he asked me to stop taking ibuprofen and instead to take a double dose of prescription-strength Nexium™. For the next six weeks, I proceeded to lose focus and to lose weight, about 25 pounds! There was still no let-up to the pain. This was too much for me. During the second visit to the gastroenterologist, I pleaded with him for another test. Something about those swollen lymph nodes they had mentioned in the CAT scan some weeks ago when I first went to the hospital. He relented and agreed to recommend a PET Scan. A PET Scan is a much more detailed scan than a CAT Scan, using a radioisotope to provide a more complete picture of what's going on inside of you.

In mid-May, Penny and I went back to the radiology center for my first PET scan. While waiting for the scan, my stomach hurt so badly now that I could hardly lie down. Instead, I stood up and paced. Unfortunately, the only way PET Scans are done is for the patient to lie down. For the next twenty minutes, I would be on my back. When the time came to do the scan, I lay on the bed of the machine wriggling in pain as they slowly glided me into the chamber. "Be still now," the male nurse kept reminding me over the speaker. "Please don't move," he repeated. Every second felt like a minute, every minute like an hour. The nurse spoke to me over the speaker in the tube again reminding me not to move. *I can't take much more of this*, I thought.

Finally, it was time to glide back out. It turns out that during the scan, the nurse had seen some things that needed immediate attention. I did not know this at the time, but apparently, he was so distraught that he called the doctor right after the scan to inform him that *he could see the tumors in my body growing while he was doing the scan!* Of course, he doesn't tell me any of this. I found out about this when I went to visit my gastroenterologist a few days later. The gastroenterologist sheepishly tells me he can't help me. "You need to see someone else." He recommends a friend of his who is an oncologist. My cynical mind thinks that this seems like a referral racket. I decline the referral and walk out.

In the parking lot, I decided to call my primary care physician immediately. *I should have done this in the very beginning*, I thought to myself. My primary care physician, Dr. James, recommended an oncologist whom I immediately called. The doctor he recommended was not available the day after Memorial Day which was the next day that I could see anyone. I asked for the next available doctor, thinking that this practice was the best one to go to and any doctor there should be good. I met with Dr. Robert the following Tuesday morning.

As we go through my journey, you need to understand things from God's perspective. I hope that this will encourage you, not discourage you. I'll use different versions or translations like the King James Version (KJV), the New American Standard Bible (NASB), the Complete Jewish Bible (CJB), and The Message Bible (MSG) among other translations. To help you to better understand how we often miss God's perspective, let's first look at a passage in the gospel of John from The Message Bible (MSG). The Message Bible is easy to read and this will give you a good overview of this passage in the gospel of John.

John 9:1-9 MSG [1]*Walking down the street, Jesus saw a man blind from birth.* [2]*His disciples asked, "Rabbi, who sinned: this man or his parents, causing him to be born blind?"* [3]*Jesus said, "You're asking the wrong question. You're looking for someone to blame. There is no such cause-effect here. Look instead for what God can do.* [4]*We need to be energetically at work for the One who sent me here, working while the sun shines. When night falls, the workday is over.* [5]*For as long as I am in the world, there is plenty of light. I am the world's Light."* [6]*He said this and then spit in the dust, made a clay paste with the saliva, rubbed the paste on the blind man's eyes,* [7]*and said, "Go, wash at the Pool of Siloam" (Siloam means "Sent"). The man went and washed—and saw.* [8]*Soon the town was buzzing. His relatives and those who year after year had seen him as a blind man begging, were saying, "Why, isn't this the man we knew, who sat here and begged?"* [9]*Others said, "It's him all right!" But others objected, "It's not the same man at all. It just looks like him." He said, "It's me, the very one."*

I was dying, and, in that kind of situation, it's quite easy to focus on your circumstances. You can get caught up in the measurements and statistics of what is happening. To deal with this, I had to focus on God. I had to focus on His promises for me. I couldn't focus on my circumstances because my circumstance was very bleak. In the beginning, I wondered so many times, *"How did I get here?"* But it's distracting to do this. In the passage above, the disciples ask, "who sinned?" They ask this because it's natural for people, anyone, including a disciple, to ask this question. It's understanding the cause and effect. If there is a problem then there must be a cause, and if there's this, then there must be that. We all do this. So, it was only natural for Jesus's disciples to think there had to be some reason why this guy was blind. But Jesus turned their hearts towards compassion and asked them to look at God, not at the man and not at his illness and not at the cause of the illness. Look at God. Look for what He can do. Don't look at the problem, look at God who will deliver you from the problem.

As you go through life, voices are directing you one way or another. In the flesh, these voices aren't always perfect. Some are good, but many are not. Some of these voices are in positions of religious authority, and if you rely on what they say, you can be distracted from only looking at Jesus. As a result, you can end up focusing on yourself, on how good you are, or perhaps, how good you aren't. To receive your healing from God, you need to focus only on Jesus. God sent His Son, the Messiah, to show us what God would be like in the flesh. This Messiah pointed to God as you would expect the Messiah would do. "Look for what God can do," Jesus directed them. Like Jesus, be preoccupied with what God can do. Don't get caught up in the blame game or in knowing why things happened. It happened. Now let's let Jesus, the Messiah, deal with it.

Allow me to draw your attention to the New King James Version (NKJV) of this very same passage. In the original manuscripts, there is no punctuation. Punctuation marks are devoid of spiritual authority. Let's take this same passage and look at it in the NKJV.

> *John 9:2-5 (NKJV)* [2]*And His disciples asked Him, saying, "Rabbi, who sinned, this man or his parents, that he was born blind?"* [3]*Jesus answered, "Neither this man nor his parents sinned, but that the works of God should be revealed in him.* [4]*"I must work the works of Him who sent Me while it is day; the night is coming when no one can work.* [5]*"As long as I am in the world, I am the light of the world."*

Reading this as it is punctuated leads you to believe that God put illness on this person for some divine purpose. That's just not true. It is not God's way. God wants to heal you.

Let's now read this passage, changing only the punctuation. We'll change a comma in verse 3 and put a period there instead and meld two verses together. We'll do the same for verse 4. **Remember, we're not going to change a single word in the NKJV translation, only the punctuation.** You can easily check this by comparing the above with what we have below. Same words, different punctuation.

> John 9:2-5 (NKJV) *²And His disciples asked Him, saying, "Rabbi, who sinned, this man or his parents, that he was born blind?" ³Jesus answered, "Neither this man nor his parents sinned.*
>
> *But that the works of God should be revealed in him ⁴I must work the works of Him who sent Me while it is day.*
>
> *The night is coming when no one can work. ⁵As long as I am in the world, I am the light of the world."*

I didn't add a single word or subtract a single word to this passage in the NKJV. I only changed the punctuation which is never in the original texts. The first passage in the NKJV with the punctuation implies God brings illness for His purpose. The second passage with the same NKJV words but with the punctuation changed doesn't imply God brings illness at all. The only thing that changed was the punctuation. The second passage focuses on the good works of God through Jesus Christ.

Now, I want you to consider this from God's perspective. Jesus revealed God and showed people what God's heart was like. Jesus was God in the flesh. He took on the form of a person so that you could see how much He wants to relate to you. As a man, He spoke only what God told Him to speak. **Jesus never brought sickness on folks. Neither does God**. Jesus, the Messiah, healed everyone who came to Him for healing. He never said, "you need a little more illness to teach you humility" or "I have destined you to be full of sickness for my glory". He never once said, "You need a little more cancer to grow closer to me", or "you need to wait until you've ____" (you fill in the blanks here). Never! If you hear this in a church, never, ever go to that church again. Never! **This is not God's way.** But because we don't understand God, and we don't know how to receive from God, we say things or do things that are contrary to God's word.

Sometimes you will hear people say things like, "you need to be right with God" or "your works will produce good things for you" and other such phrases. These are not true, and they do not line up with God's word. Usually, this way of thinking is taught to us by those in positions of religious authority who don't themselves understand the word and the heart of God. Contrary to what you may have been taught, God's true heart is as a Shepherd to us.

Don't Wrestle with It, Rest in It.

We live in a new covenant. Jesus died for you and me, not just to take away our sins, but to give us His gift of righteousness too. In other words, Jesus died to make sure that you are always right with God. God doesn't have anything against you anymore. All your sins were paid for in a just manner, and that includes yesterday's sins, today's sins, and tomorrow's sins. God is a just God and He has already demanded punishment for them in the body of His Son, our Messiah. In the Old Covenant, he reminded his people year after year that sins must be paid for or atoned for. That's why they celebrated a Day of Atonement. But when the Messiah came, He paid for it all, once and for all time. His work on the cross is a complete, finished work. Nothing is lacking in what Jesus Christ did for us. You don't have to pay for your sins again because Jesus paid for them *in full* about 2000 years ago. I say this so that you will not think in your heart that your illness is some punishment from God.

Sickness is not from God. Get that in your head and get it in your heart. Your life depends on believing this truth. Jesus, the Messiah, is our Redeemer. He purchased for us complete forgiveness of sins, freedom from shame, freedom from lack, and freedom from depression. His last words on the cross tell you that it's over. You don't have to pay anything more to get His peace, His provision, His love, or His healing for you. His last words on the cross were, "*It is finished.*" You just need to *rest* in that truth. Don't wrestle with it, *rest* in it. Believe it. He became a curse for us so that we would no longer live a cursed life.

You have hope! It's in Jesus Christ, not in you, not in medicine, not in doctors, not in vegetables, and not in vitamins. While many of these things are good for you, they do not compare to what Jesus *already* provided for you at the cross. He's got this. You are not defeated. When the sick came to Jesus, He always healed them. Don't be afraid. And don't let your heart be troubled.

3.

AT DEATH'S DOOR

During my first visit to my oncologist, Dr. Robert, he revealed that he could not confirm cancer of any kind without a biopsy. It was obvious at that point that I was in a very weak state after being misdiagnosed and treated for an ulcer for the past six weeks. Time wasn't waiting for me. We discussed what would happen if cancer were confirmed with a biopsy. A biopsy requires surgery. After this surgery, I would then need to have a second surgical procedure done to put a port into my right shoulder area so that chemo could be administered. Only then could I go to the hospital for chemotherapy. "Doctor, can we speed up this process? I'm concerned with how long this will take," I asked Dr. Robert. He agreed to check with a surgeon friend of his to see if he could combine both procedures in one surgery. After waiting for two days, which seemed like an eternity, I received the confirmation that both procedures could and would be done by his colleague. I would go to a hospital within the next few days.

Ok, this is serious, I'm thinking. *But I don't need, and I don't want anyone causing my wife to panic.* My wife and I feed off each other's strengths. I love so much that Penny will allow me to say what the word of God says and leave it as is. She doesn't add her conditions

or qualifications. It is "amen" to the word of God. She is such a
blessing to me this way. I decided to post something on my church's
Facebook page that I'm sure most of my friends were shocked to
read. I don't remember my exact words, but it was something like
the following:

> Dear church friends, I am going to be hospitalized
> and I need your prayers. However, I don't want you to pray
> for my healing. Healing is already promised to me in the
> bible because it says, "by Jesus Christ's stripes you have been
> healed." But I need your prayers for physical and spiritual
> strength. I don't know what I must go through, but I know
> I will need this.

After I posted this, I shut down my computer and moved to our
bedroom to lay down and rest. I would not touch my computer
again until I was released from the hospital. It felt better to rest and
just let it go. I was not going to fight this thing anymore. I couldn't.
This was not my battle to fight. Plus, I didn't have a lot of strength,
so I needed to conserve whatever little I had left for the days that
lay ahead.

A few days after the surgery to put my port in, which required a
hospital overnight stay, I was back in Dr. Robert's office with Penny.
We discussed his findings from the biopsy. He explained to us that I
had an aggressive form of cancer. Burkitt's-like, he explained, which
simply means that it was aggressive and spreading quickly. I had
just been diagnosed with non-Hodgkin's-Lymphoma. Dr. Robert
assured me that it was treatable but because it was an aggressive
form, we didn't have time to waste. I needed to go into the hospital
in a few days where I would need to go through four cycles of
chemotherapy, each cycle lasting about 7 weeks long. The thought
occurred to me that I was hurtling toward death and needed to
put the brakes on the progress of this cancer. Unbeknownst to me

at the time, because I don't usually focus on Doctor reports, the results of a FISH (Florescence in situ hybridization) test showed the following "This is an ABNORMAL result (all caps was put in by the lab physician) and is an evidence of "Triple Hit Lymphoma." Per a search on Google, I found the following: *Triple-hit lymphoma is a rare but serious form of Non-Hodgkin's lymphoma that is known to have a worse prognosis than diffuse large B-cell lymphoma (DLBCL) or Burkitt lymphoma (BL) alone, with a survival time of only a few months.* This search was done on Oct 27, 2015.

A few days later, Penny and I went back to Dr. Robert's office for one last visit to review my situation with his colleagues. I didn't realize at the time that I may only have about a month or so to live. I am grateful to Dr. Robert for not describing it this way to me and my wife. To me, that was compassion on his part. Dr. Robert called over two other doctors and asked them for their recommendations. I remember sitting on the examining table, my shoulders heavy with weakness. Time had taken its toll on me and I was in a very weak state. I wandered in and out of focus and I could hardly pay attention while sitting there. My legs dangled beneath me while the two doctors stood at the end of the examining table talking to each other. One of them was a seasoned doctor. The other, Dr. Julia, was a relatively new doctor who specializes in these types of cancers. I didn't understand what they were saying to each other, so I just worked on pacing myself. "*One step at a time, Phil,*" I tell myself. "*If I don't move too fast, I'll get through this.*" But the reality was that I had no real fight left in me, only the fight to take the next breath, one breath at a time. The two doctors continued speaking to each other in their foreign medical language. Occasionally, they glanced up at me with faint, polite smiles.

I'm a dead man, I think. *I am just a specimen to them. I am just someone in a petri dish who needs to be doused or prodded or sprinkled with chemo dust to ascertain what the reaction will be.* But my fight in that office before these physicians was to focus and look like I was mentally sharp so that I could manage to ask a few meaningful questions. My speech was slow, deliberate, and thoughtful. I didn't want the doctors thinking poorly of me. It was silly for me to think this way.

After what seemed like a few hours of what was probably just a few minutes, the doctors turned to us and tried to explain their treatment plan to me and Penny. They used technical terms I did not understand. *I really don't care,* I think. *I'm fighting for my life here. What is the next step? What do I do next?* I didn't want them dismissing me as some hopeless cause, so I pretended to listen and engage. I didn't have any strength to fight this in any other way. Even this approach seemed to be too much. I let out a big sigh. Tired, I pushed to stay focused on what they were saying. The doctors finished by telling me they wanted to call an ambulance to take me to the hospital even though the hospital was within walking distance, just two minutes away by car. With a blood pressure of 70/50, they didn't think that I'd make it to the hospital on my own. So, very, very slowly, Penny and I walked to the front of the office building where the ambulance was already waiting. The ambulance crew put me on the gurney and as they lifted me to put me in the back of the ambulance, I could feel every bump of the metal gurney and blacked-out.

I woke up to find myself slumped over in a wheelchair in the waiting area of the emergency room of the hospital. I was fighting with everything within me to not blackout again, *Just one moment at a time, Phil,* I tell myself. *Breathe in, breathe out.* A friend from my past came to the emergency room and noticed me, he was working at the hospital as an orderly. I couldn't speak to him. It took too much energy. I was dying. I needed every ounce of energy for this fight. I smiled faintly to acknowledge him, but I was speechless. My wife explained everything to him. I had no energy to add to what she was saying. *Can we continue this discussion some other time?* I thought, somewhat impatiently. He prayed for me and mentioned that he'd visit me later in the week.

Another friend came by. Jess was an acquaintance from a church my wife and I were attending at the time. He had come over from another wing of the hospital across the street. How Jess heard about my being there, I have no idea, but I was glad he was there. I later learned that his wife had been in the other wing having just given birth to a beautiful baby boy. Jess had his characteristic big smile and talked with me, but he did not really expect me to carry on a deep conversation. As a marine sergeant, Jess knew better. He knew how to take charge. He immediately began praying for me. His prayer was strong, not weak. Direct. He reminded God of His promises to us. Then he emptied a small bottle of oil on my head. The whole bottle was dumped on my head! In one sense, it was funny. In another sense, it was bold. But I didn't care anymore. I didn't let it bother me. He prayed over me and, just as Sergeant Jess finished his prayer, a nurse came in, looked at him, and then at me, then back at Jess again. "Oh, we were just anointing him with oil and praying over him," Jess barked out with a big smile. The nurse wiped the oil from my forehead. She'd probably seen all kinds of kooks in the emergency room. Another day, another kook, she was probably thinking. This time I blacked out for good. The next time I was awake was in the intensive care unit several days later.

Sometimes, crises will reveal to you who you are. My wife, Penny, showed herself to be strong toward God when this stuff hit the fan. She went back home later that evening and had holy communion, reminding God, and reminding herself, that Jesus did not die in vain. "*By His stripes, I was healed,*" she confessed aloud and alone. But in times like this, you need someone to walk beside you, to lift you up with encouragement, to let you know that your hope is not in vain. I thank God for my pastor at that time, Pastor Aaron. We had first come to the church about 7 months earlier. It was a young church that was growing rapidly under his enthusiastic leadership. Here was a pastor who was excited about God's word and, more than that, about Jesus Christ. My wife spoke to him and, I'm sure, he pushed aside his doubts and any doubts my wife may have had, by bringing the focus back to God's faithfulness. What do you say in a situation like this? I am so grateful he chose to simply say the word of God rather than some pious platitude about grinning and bearing it. He brought the focus back to God and what He could do.

Later, I would learn that he went to his pastor, who was also a mentor to him, for counsel. After seeing me in my condition, Pastor Aaron was shaken and felt that he might need to prepare my wife and counsel her for my death. However, in his discussions with his mentor, he remarked on how I was only confessing what God's word said, not what the doctor's reports revealed. The mentor's counsel to this pastor of mine was simple, *"let him have what he says."* I am so thankful for this wise counsel to my pastor. Pastor Aaron came back a few days later with Jess and they left me with a book of promises to confess over myself as I went through this ordeal. The book contained bible verses that were encouraging and uplifting. After they left the booklet with me, they left my room shaken by what they had seen. I was not aware of this at the time, but, according to them, I looked so bad to them that they spent the next 10-15 minutes in concentrated prayer for me in the lobby of the hospital.

The next few days in intensive care were a blur. I couldn't tell one day from the next or how long I had been there as I drifted in and out of consciousness usually awake for just a few minutes before sliding back off to sleep. The few times that I was awake, I played a scenario in my head where I had teamed up with Clint Eastwood and we discussed a movie plot. My voice, now turned gravely because of the tumors around my throat area, reminded me of Clint Eastwood when I talked out aloud. But I have tumors everywhere. Over and over, I thought, *"how did I get here?"*

4.

MY BARGAINING NATURE KICKS IN

My first conscious moments interacting with others that I can remember is Father's Day! My children came to visit me in the hospital, along with two of my future sons-in-law. I'm sure they had probably come to visit before, but I don't remember. I have three of the most wonderful daughters in the world. Each so different from the other. Julia, my oldest, does not care to see pain, especially the pain of a loved one. She is very direct about this and because we are frank with each other, I completely understand. Occasionally, she would come by with Ken, her boyfriend at the time, and now my son-in-law. Ken is easy-going and non-judgmental. This helped Julia manage this confrontation with death that I was going through. I didn't feel slighted in the least because she didn't come by to visit very much. I understood her needs. I love my children dearly and I know and understand their differences.

Laura, my middle child, on the other hand, made a conscious effort to "be present with me." She too is non-judgmental and is gifted with a listening heart. She walks with a "presence" or an "awareness" of you. She would ask how I was handling things and I would respond with what happened and what the concerns were.

Sometimes she just didn't know what to do. With a strong internal character, she simply and patiently sat with me, not expecting anything in return. But in her own words, this is how she characterized seeing me: She very vividly remembers me looking like a skeleton or a baby (an ugly one :-)) or even an alien! To her, my eyes were yellow, veiny, and bulging unnaturally while the rest of my body and face was deathly sunken in, and my whole frame was so skinny except for the tumors on my stomach area. I looked extremely near dying to her and I'm sure I looked this way to everyone else. I can only imagine that I was frightening to look at and this was even more terrifying in my daughter's mind.

Alyson, my youngest, springs into action. Living in Austin, TX at the time, she immediately arranged to come to our home to be with her mom and to visit me. She works out of her home in Austin and was able to work out of our home in Florida during my hospital stay. Alyson is not afraid to cry when she needs to. She wants to communicate the fullness of what she is experiencing. She is a good listener too. We had some good cries together when she visited.

I never wanted to look at myself, so when I went to the bathroom, I avoided the mirror. I only took two pictures of myself during this first cycle of chemo. To see myself was to look at my circumstances and it would magnify them over what I knew was in the word of God. It bothered me that my children had to see me in this state, but at least I was not looking at me. I was focused on the promises of my loving Lord and Savior. To do otherwise would have been to enter despair. I'm sure my children were frightened that their Dad could leave them at any minute and leave life in this manner. I am so blessed that none of them, including my wife, said anything about how I looked. It would have made me more conscious of my dire circumstances.

Father's Day that year was a long, exhausting day for me. My wife wanted me to get out in the sun thinking the vitamin D would do me some good. She cleared this with the nursing staff, and we prepared to get some sun. Early that afternoon, we went out to the patio where the hot Florida sun awaited us. I had lost a lot of weight and the warm sun melted away my body chills while sitting in my wheelchair. The heat felt so good. But my children were sweating, and I sensed this, so we didn't stay too long on the hospital deck. After all, it was June and Florida summers can be sweltering.

After we came back to my hospital room, my children stayed to chat briefly. The fog was clearing, and I was starting to remember things. I remembered Ephesians chapter 6 where it says, "*honor your father and mother for this is the first commandment with a promise.*" I wanted to live, and this was a promise with a condition attached to it. My father had died only a year before, and now, laying in the hospital bed, it was all coming back to me. I was remembering all of this and imagining how I could've honored my father better. As I reflected on my life as a son, I realized that I had not always honored my father in the past. I had often complained to my girls about my father when they were growing up. Sometimes, I had even criticized him in front of them. I knew in my heart that it wasn't right. It wasn't honoring my dad. My father and I didn't see eye to eye in most things and we had struggled in our relationship for most of my teen and early adult years. I loved him, but I needed him to love me back, to openly and unabashedly say he loved me. However, he was both a World War II and a Korean War vet, and those guys just don't do that. Because I had often talked unkindly about my father, I realized that I hadn't been the greatest example in the world to my kids when it came to showing them how to honor their father.

Guilt welled up inside me and I began to tell my kids how much my dad meant to me on this Father's Day. I brought up my father so often that Julia, my oldest daughter, astutely noticed and asked me why I was focusing on my dad and not on myself on Father's Day. I love Julia's openness. I think she knew without coming right out and saying it. She is like her mom this way and I so appreciated her noticing this.

It was time to make amends, and even though my father was no longer alive, I knew that the way forward was to show God that I was repenting and changing my mind and that I wanted to set an example for my children. I didn't want to give God any reason not to give me a longer life. I wanted to show my children that when you honor your parents, He'll give you a long life. For me, sixty years wasn't nearly long enough. I wanted more. I knew they would have children and I wanted to enjoy seeing their children.

I did the only thing I knew to do at that time, which was to honor my father because I wanted to hold on to that promise which carried a long life[2]. But what I was doing was bargaining with God in my weak state. If "I" do this, then "you'll" give me a long life. It's a quid-pro-quo. I didn't want to tell Julia or my other children that I felt like I was dying because I thought this might scare them. But I knew within myself that it was a intensely serious time in my life.

I didn't know how I was going to get out of this predicament called cancer. I felt very weak, and the possibility of death had become real to me. I stuffed away any fear I had about cancer, especially in front of my children. Sometimes, I would console myself by thinking, *"well, in one hundred years or one thousand years, it will not make a difference because all of my loved ones would be with me*

---

[2] Ephesians 6:2-3 (NASB) *2HONOR YOUR FATHER AND MOTHER (which is the first commandment with a promise), 3SO THAT IT MAY BE WELL WITH YOU, AND THAT YOU MAY LIVE LONG ON THE EARTH.*

This is taken from the following Old Testament verse. That's why it's in ALL CAPS. It's not a mistake on the part of the author and it's not God shouting at you. It's the way most versions show that this is quoted from the Old Testament. In Deuteronomy 5:16 (NASB) it says, '*Honor your father and your mother, as the LORD your God has commanded you, that your days may be prolonged and that it may go well with you on the land which the LORD your God gives you.*

in heaven and I wouldn't need to be afraid." But this fear was real. Maybe it wasn't outright fear, but the thought loomed in my mind that I could be dead soon, within weeks, if not within the next few days.

As I said earlier, Father's Day was exhausting. It was too much to attend to each person and to myself. When you're deathly ill, it is a fight to be pleasant and social and to "entertain" guests, even if they are blood family. I would recommend caregivers, and those who are caring for those who are struggling with treatments for cancer or some other serious illness, to give 'alone time' to your loved one. Give them 'rest time'. They need physical rest. To be away from noise and distractions. It's not that they don't want to spend time with you, it's just that it takes a lot of energy to spend time with you. My children left and I napped for the rest of the afternoon.

When I awoke later that evening, I watched the fifth game of the NBA finals between the Houston Rockets and the Miami Heat. My children had mentioned during their afternoon visit that the game would be on TV later that evening. Bret, Alyson's boyfriend at the time and now my son-in-law, was not too happy with the results thus far. He told me it could boil down to this final fifth game. I watched the game with relief and anticipation. It was so exciting to finally feel alive and to be able to cheer on the Houston Rockets! They won the NBA finals that night on June 15th, eight days after I entered the hospital. I wasn't even aware of what was going on till that final fifth game. I know I live in Florida, but the players were older on the Houston Rockets and I identified with older guys winning the NBA Finals.

5.

FALLEN FROM GRACE

When I realized how much I had dishonored my father while he was alive, I did the only thing I knew to do at that time, I tried to rectify the situation by beginning to honor him with my words. I began to undo the things I had said about him to my children. I thought I was honoring him of my own free will when all I was doing was honoring him because I wanted to hold on to God's promise which carried a long life. I was bargaining with God.

What I failed to realize was that you don't negotiate with God, He doesn't need what you have. Besides, you aren't able to give Him anything. You see, when He gave us His Son, Jesus, He more than paid for any debt you have with God. You can't pay anything compared to what Christ paid for you on the cross. His payment for your debt was full, complete, overflowing. It was more than enough! Nothing more can be paid and there can be no doubt in anyone's mind that, nothing but a full payment was made. When you are in debt to someone, the last thing you want to do is to be around that person. It just reminds you of your debt to them, so you avoid them at all costs. This is the way many people are with God. They feel that they "owe" Him because of what they have done or what they haven't done in their life. But if that debt were overpaid, say ten or one hundred times over, well you would have no problem being around that person. You'd probably expect them to take you out to lunch or dinner. After all, the debt was *overpaid.*

But if you don't look at Jesus, and instead look at yourself and think about what you can bring to the table, then you'll be guilty of the law you've set up for yourself. Get rid of all guilt by looking at Jesus and seeing that His payment for you was IN FULL. If you want to be healed, it's important to understand God's perspective on this. Don't go with the tradition of man or with the edicts of religious leadership that don't point you to Christ. As you accompany me on my journey, I'm going to share with you what I learned and how you can receive all that God wants for you.

There is no quid pro quo with God! If you do good to get good, you cut yourself off from Christ. Putting yourself under the law makes you fallen from grace! We read in Galatians 5:4 (King James Version) that "Christ is become of no effect unto you, whosoever of you are justified by the law; ye are fallen from grace."

Under the law, you can't draw near to Him. You won't come to Him until you feel, in your mind and heart, that you are guilt-free before Him. But you can't pay for your sins or your redemption or your healing. It's a gift wrapped up in Jesus Christ in *His finished work* on the cross. He took everything on Himself, all judgment, all pain, all sickness, and disease so you wouldn't have any. He gave you the gift of righteousness, which is rightness before God, also sometimes called right standing with God. You see, when you are right with someone, you can ask them anything. You're not imposing on them and you're not timid with them. You know you are *right* with them.

Romans 10:4 (ESV) "*For Christ is the end of the law for righteousness to everyone who believes.*"

2 Corinthians 5:21 (ESV) *"For our sake he made him to be sin who knew no sin, so that in him we might become the righteousness of God."*

This righteousness depends on Jesus, *not* on the right things *you do*, however noble the things you do may seem in your own eyes.

Sin doesn't separate you from God, depending on you does. In Galatians 5:4 (NIV) we read: *You who are trying to be justified by law have been alienated from Christ; you have fallen away from grace.* Think of rules and regulations. That's the law. If you are trying to be justified by your good works, you have fallen from grace. Think of grace as a person, Jesus the Christ. If you justify yourself by your works, you alienate yourself from the Messiah who is your healer. Instead, believe in the Lord Jesus Christ, that God raised Him from the dead to give you His righteousness. In other words, Jesus gave you *His rightness with God.* This is what you "step into," Christ and His righteousness. You are right with God because of Jesus, never because of your good works! Sin doesn't separate you from God, depending on your works does, even if they are good works. When I was bargaining with God, I was depending on my works, my performance for Him. I didn't realize or act on the truth that I am forgiven for sins I have committed, sins I was committing, and sins I will commit. Past, present, and future. They were all future sins at the cross. Falling from grace is not some great sin as a natural man would have you believe. Falling from grace is simply putting yourself under the works of the law to be right before God. It's like saying Jesus the Messiah wasn't good enough and what you do will make it good enough. When you do this, you alienate or separate yourself from Christ your healer, and you are fallen from grace.

But in the back of my mind in that hospital room, I felt I needed to deserve my healing. To be worthy enough in God's eyes to receive my healing. That's why I bargained with God. It doesn't work. God gives without reproach. He gives now more than ever because His Son, the Messiah, has satisfied His need for judgment. My blessings from Him are now free. 1 Corinthians 2:12 (NIV) says, *We have not received the spirit of the world but the Spirit who is from God, that we may understand what God **has freely given** us*[3]. The Jewish notion of God is of a deity who wants to bless His people, that no curse alights on them from God. We have this same God. A God who wants to bless us "in Christ." "In Christ" is every blessing that we have in life. It is His Shalom we are given. Shalom is peace with God, peace with your neighbors, peace with your demands and, therefore, no lack. "My Shalom I give to you", Christ said in the gospels. Romans 8:32 (NIV) says *He who did not spare his own Son, but gave him up for us all—how will he not also, along with him, **graciously give us all things**?* This is a rhetorical question to get us to think. He loved us so much that He didn't spare His own Son. Who would give up their only son for anything? God loved the Messiah, His Son, so much, yet He gave Him up for us. That tells you how much He loves you! His Son was good. You and I are not good, even on our best days. The very next verses of Romans tell us that we are not condemned by God.

Romans 8:33-35 (NIV) *Who will bring any charge against those whom God has chosen? It is God who justifies.*

---

[3] When I quote scripture, **Bold** is my emphasis. There is no punctual authority in the word of God. So commas, periods, and my **bolded** words have no divine authority. It's just my emphasis, that's all.

Who is he that condemns? Christ Jesus, who died—more than that, who was raised to life—is at the right hand of God and is also interceding for us. Who shall separate us from the love of Christ? Shall trouble or hardship or persecution or famine or nakedness or danger or sword?

Who will bring any charge against those whom God has chosen? No one! It is God who justifies you. Justification is the same thing as righteousness. You are right before God. His Son is interceding for you now, not when you feel He is! Even when we sin, He is interceding with God on our behalf. Is there anything that would separate us from the love of God in Christ? No. Now, let's look at 2 Peter.

2 Peter 1:2-4 (ESV) "²May grace and peace be multiplied to you in the knowledge of God and of Jesus our Lord. ³His divine power has granted to us all things that pertain to life and godliness, through the knowledge of him who called us to his own glory and excellence, ⁴by which he has granted to us his precious and very great promises, so that through them you may become partakers of the divine nature, having escaped from the corruption that is in the world because of sinful desire."

He "has", past tense, given us everything we need for life and godliness. How was this given? Through knowing the One, the Messiah, the Christ! Keep your focus on Christ. He is your healer. Keep your heart beating with knowing that He ONLY has good intentions for you. Forget what some religious leader may have told you about working to earn or deserve God's love and blessings. There are no five steps to deliverance or three steps to a better relationship with God, etc. These are man-made constructs that take your focus away from the Lord Jesus Christ with self-righteous works that are designed to make us focus on us. God's love and God's blessings are already yours in Christ! *You only need to learn how to take these blessings* and you do that by focusing on Him, by simply looking at Him.

6.

HEALING ISN'T SURVIVING!

I was supposed to go through four cycles of chemotherapy. Each cycle was to be approximately seven to eight weeks long! While going through the first cycle, I wondered how I was supposed to last long enough for three more cycles. I thought to myself, *I could die from this*! And if I didn't die right away, what would my lifestyle be like after four cycles of chemo?

In those early days in the hospital, I didn't know what was going on, and I was still in much pain. My wife and I were determined that God would provide a way out of this misery. At this point, I wasn't thinking of being healed, instead, I was thinking of getting out of the hospital. My trust wasn't directed to God, instead I was trying to scheme my way through getting out of the hospital. My wife and I just didn't know what or how this would be done. I mean, was I supposed to walk out of the hospital after ripping out the IVs from my arms? For the most part, I was not afraid except for those first eight to ten days when I felt within myself that this could be the end of my life. During the "first cycle" of chemo that lasted seven weeks, my life became a routine of daily medicines punctuated with minor adjustments based on my observed condition, or the stats my body provided.

I needed lots of medicine, and the doctor's determined that my port wasn't enough. A port is an object that was put on my right side just below my collarbone. It was surgically placed to allow medicine into the body through a tube that goes into a vein in your chest and ultimately ends up at your heart. It's under the skin, but there is a small silver dollar-sized plastic piece that sticks out on the outside of your body. This is where they connect tubes for the medicine and for the chemo to pass through to the rest of your body.

But even a port wasn't enough given how sick I was. The port was in use full-time and yet I needed more. To supplement the port, the doctors determined in those first few days that I needed a PICC line inserted in my left arm in addition to the port on my right side. A PICC line is a long tube that is inserted into a vein in your arm or sometimes into a vein in your leg. Like the port, it allows medicines to get into a large vein that goes to the heart.

Occasionally, temporary nurses would fill in if someone were on vacation or out for some other reason. One such nurse took care of me the day I had my PICC line put in. Life can be rough if you're being shuttled from one station to the next, so I usually tried to strike up a conversation with each person I met to make the journey as pleasant as possible for everyone. If I were nice to them, perhaps they'd be nice to me (notice that my bargaining nature pops up everywhere). Sometimes in their conversations, they'll give you a little background on themselves. I can't remember the name of my temporary nurse, so I'll call her Lola. Lola was a small Argentinian beauty who knew she was a looker. She was usually sticking needles into me for one reason or another and she liked to flirt. I had just turned 60 and I'm sure I looked more like I was 90. In my condition, what was I supposed to do? Lola would tap the needle, swirl her hair to the right, arch her back, and give the needle a small squirt so there wouldn't be pockets of air in the needle. I think she liked to do this in front of me. This lady was all show, and I had a ringside seat.

Lola was the one who accompanied me down to the surgery area to get the PICC line inserted. The area was on the bottom floor of the hospital where it is coldest. To prepare me for the procedure, they moved me to a cold hard surface. I'd lost considerable weight by then and every bone in my back felt that cold board. I needed an ultrasound on the arm to ensure the vein was large enough and to ensure that they could find a spot to put the PICC line in. Dr. Leah was listening to rock music blaring in the background while focusing on the ultrasound. The ultrasound would tell her where to put the PICC line. Dr. Leah and Lola were chatting it up when Lola suggested that they change the music to heavy metal. It's not like I'm deaf, I could hear everything. I was not sedated. The whole process, the loud music, and the banter was making me incredibly anxious. I asked God to work with Dr. Leah to give her the wisdom to do this procedure correctly.

I watched as she struggled with the PICC line placement and had to pull it out and try again. At that point, I began to pray with even more intensity that God would take over because Dr. Leah surely couldn't figure out where this PICC line needed to go. I should have demanded that the music be turned off, but I was acting nice as a bargaining boy should. *"If I'm nice to them, they'll be nice to me"*, I thought. It didn't work. The doctor seemed clueless about finding the vein. Weeks later I would develop an infection at that very spot that ultimately led to several surgeries on my left hand to remove fungal infections. Finally, on the second attempt, the PICC line was correctly set up. I was as tense as can be. But it was over. At least for that event. I let go, relaxed, and slept like a baby when they brought me back to my room. I think I slept until the next day because I was so exhausted from the tense exercise and the danger I had gone through.

Each day, new "events" were taking place. I wasn't panicking, but these events were requiring me to quietly steel my mind against the forces that were coming at me. *"Forget the past, don't think ahead. Focus on the now,"* I kept telling myself. I was depending on my calmness to carry me through but that was silly. Calmness doesn't get you healed, and it won't make going through something like this any easier. I needed healing. How do I receive the healing that God says He made available to me 2000+ years ago in the finished work of Jesus Christ? What button do I need to push to get this healing that's promised to me? At this point, it was all about me and my actions. I wasn't even thinking about receiving healing from God. I was thinking about what I needed to do, not who provided my healing.

Fluid had been building up in my body and the doctors overseeing my care determined that I was strong enough to get the fluid removed from my lungs. Every day, I felt like I was on the brink of falling off the cliff of life and into death's chasm. One of the doctors working with the cancer team came to my room and casually stated that I had too much fluid in my lungs and they needed to remove it. "It won't hurt," he said, trying to sound reassuring.

I was prepared to head back down to the basement of the hospital, *where many go to die in their last battle of life*, I think. I had to be awake for this procedure. *"Great"*, I thought to myself, *"just what I need."* They'd go in from the back with a long needle into my lungs to draw out the fluid, in this case, a whopping 1.5 liters of fluid! On top of this, I was also due for a spinal tap. I tried to talk myself through it because I knew that even if I got through this 'right now' moment, there would still be later 'right now' moments to deal with. I told myself not to lose energy because *"you can't control everything."* I really can't control anything, but I'm not thinking this way. I stay quiet, focused, and living, in the right now. I lay very still for the spinal tap. One wrong move and I shuddered to think of the consequences. They numbed the area where the needle would go in. *Be still now.* I feel a sharp, cold pinch. *"That's it. Be still Phil,"* I tell myself. How long can this last? Twenty minutes later the procedure ended. My chest heaves a sigh of relief. I long to go to sleep to forget these daily traumas.

Throughout these events, I was looking to be "able" to persist through my will power. My focus was on lasting through each episode long enough to get to the next one. 1st Corinthians 2:12 (NASB) says, *"Now we have received, not the spirit of the world, but the Spirit who is from God, so that we may know the things **freely given to us by God.**"* My mind wasn't on God and I wasn't looking to Him for His strength. It was on me and my abilities and my strength. It was instinctive and natural to consider what I could do for my situation. Most times, I couldn't do anything except to be still. Instead, my thought should have turned to God and His ability for me. God wants us to know what *He's freely* given to us. God wants us to *be aware of His ability* instead of our ability. Focusing on God and His ability enables you to only see victory for yourself. You relax better. You don't have to know the details. ***You just trust that He is faithful to His word.*** Only later during this seven-week ordeal, would I put my focus on my Savior, Jesus Christ.

To be focused on God's goodness, on God's faithfulness, on God's ability, and not your goodness, you need to feed on the word of God. You need to hear messages about who you are in Christ and what He has done for you with one sacrifice for all time on the cross. I didn't even read my bible during this time. It was too much work for me. When I read my bible, I prefer to study the word. I had no energy for studying. As I gained physical strength, I turned to the teaching of Pastor Joseph Prince, reading one of his books, *The Power of Right Believing*. But not in the beginning. I was simply too weak.

Once I started to focus on God alone, I understood that God loves me and only wants to bless me *with no strings attached*. I want you to see Him as only wanting you healed. If you know something is freely given to you, you can **take it freely.** Don't be embarrassed to take it. Just take it. Fix in your mind and your heart that His blessings are for you and they are for the taking. Get a mindset to take from God. Take what is freely given to you.

You can't see this if you are focusing on what you need to do for God or on what you need to give God. If your mind is thinking about the price you must pay, you will never take what's rightfully yours. You are stuck in an old covenant mindset. But God's promises, because of the finished work of His Son, weren't rightfully yours because of your goodness or because of your good effort. It's rightfully yours because of Jesus Christ and the work He said He completed ("*finished*") at the cross. It's rightfully yours because of your faith in Jesus Christ and what Christ did, once and for all. This is a new covenant mindset. One that recognizes that Jesus *finished* the work He came to accomplish, that He was a perfect sacrifice, so you don't even have to try to be a good sacrifice. You just take what's *freely given* to you. **You bless God by taking from Him what He's always wanted to give to you.**

Is God Willing? I Know He's Able.

Even though I had many problems in the way I approached God in the beginning, I knew that He wanted me healed. Of course, I also knew that He was able to heal me. You must know and understand that God is willing and that He is able. Most times we are sure that God is able. However, we're not always so sure that He is willing. Why? Because we look at ourselves as needing to deserve it. That means you make a rule that enables you to see you deserve it. That's a state that God characterizes as fallen from grace. It is putting yourself under obligation, under law, even if it's under your law or your own rule. We've all heard of the story of Shadrach, Meshach, and Abednego. How did they respond to threats against their lives? In Daniel 3:17 (NASB) it says, "*If it be so, our God whom we serve is able to deliver us* *from the furnace of blazing fire;* *and He will* *deliver us* *out of your hand, O king."* God was able and God is willing - that's what they confessed and believed. They didn't have to know how. They just knew that He would deliver them. And they were willing to say this with their mouth. God is able. And in the new covenant, we see Jesus showing that He also is willing; not just able, but willing too.

> In Mark 1:40-42 (NASB) we read: [40]*And a leper came to Jesus, beseeching Him and falling on his knees before Him, and saying, "If You are willing, You can make me clean."* [41]*Moved with compassion, Jesus stretched out His hand and touched him, and said to him, "I am willing; be cleansed."* [42]*Immediately the leprosy left him and he was cleansed.*

When you see Jesus, you see the heart of God. When you looked at Him, you saw God. Jesus was moved with compassion. We have a compassionate God who is for us. He is willing. So much so that He reaches out and touches an unclean person to make them clean. The more you understand what God is able and willing to do, the more you will be able to trust him.

Perhaps, the leper heard the commotion in the countryside about this prophet or Messiah and all the healings He performed. But was He willing to heal him, a leper? Did God love Him enough? Did that love go so far as to heal him specifically? Or was it just a love thought with no action? After all, the leper was considered unclean. Was the leper worthy of God's love? Jesus answered it definitively. He touched him.

Oh, how He loves us. He is not afraid to touch us when we aren't perfect, when we're dirty or unclean. He wants to demonstrate His love for us. It's "how" we more than overcome in this world, through His love for us[4]. Notice what happened next. Jesus told the man to go to the priest to offer the gift that Moses commanded. What does this mean? Why did Jesus instruct him to do this? We read in Matthew 8:4 (NIV), *Then Jesus said to him, "See that you don't tell anyone. But go, show yourself to the priest and offer the gift Moses commanded, as a testimony to them."* The priest had to pronounce him clean. Why did Jesus say this? Why is this recorded in the gospel? Because today we are the priests of God through Christ in us. And we have greater power in us than the priests of the old testament because of our High Priest, Jesus the Messiah, who lives in us. In Leviticus 27:12 (NASB) we read, *'The priest shall value it as either good or bad; as you, the priest, value it, so it shall be.* You, as a priest in the new covenant, value your life as either good or bad. You pronounce yourself healed by your Savior, Jesus the Christ, the Messiah. And if you have confessed Jesus as Lord, then you pronounce yourself clean because of the blood of His Son, not because of your good works or good thoughts.

Today, everyone is talking up a storm about how we need to get clean or get rid of the junk in our lives. And while this is noble, don't put yourself under the bondage of the old covenant. Let Jesus Christ establish you and work in you to do this. The old covenant has been replaced by a new covenant of grace where we are also kings and priests. Jesus, our Messiah, is King of Kings and Lord of Lords and He is our High Priest. We pronounce ourselves clean before God just as the priest pronounced someone clean. How are you going to do that? By faith. By opening your mouth, the weakest part of your body with the most potential for power exercised. By using your eyes to look and see that Jesus wants you healed. These things aren't hard. You aren't going to look at your circumstances, instead, you're going to look at the cross and see and confess that Jesus made you clean, and that by His stripes you are healed.

---

[4] Romans 8:37 (NIV) *No, in all these things we are more than conquerors through him who loved us.*

In 1 Peter 2:9-10 (NASB) it says, [9]*But you are A CHOSEN RACE, A royal PRIESTHOOD, A HOLY NATION, A PEOPLE FOR God's OWN POSSESSION, so that you may proclaim the excellencies of Him who has called you out of darkness into His marvelous light;* [10]*for you once were NOT A PEOPLE, but now you are THE PEOPLE OF GOD; you had NOT RECEIVED MERCY, but now you have RECEIVED MERCY.*

What do Kings do? They say what they want! They declare it. And other people carry it out. So, speak forth your healing. Call yourself healed in Christ. Call cancer dead in your body. Be the priest God has made you to be in Christ. Be the king God has made you in Christ and pronounce yourself clean because of the finished work of Christ. Then watch God carry it out. You are now the people of God and you have now received His mercy. At first, I was a bit timid. I distinctly remember looking down at myself and calling cancer dead. But it was more of a whimper, not a declaration. But that's ok. You speak and sow the seed of God's word in your life.

God took on the form of a man in our Messiah for a reason. As a man, Jesus the Messiah understands what you are going through. In Hebrews 4:15-16 (NASB) we read [15]*For we do not have a high priest who cannot sympathize with our weaknesses, but One who has been tempted in all things as we are, yet without sin.* [16]*Therefore let us draw near with confidence to the throne of grace, so that we may receive mercy and find grace to help in time of need.*

Jesus is not a stranger to need. And when He is with us, He has compassion for us. He loves us tenderly and dearly. He understands rejection. He understands pain and suffering. He doesn't want you to continue to experience these things. He paid a price, once and for all so that we would no longer have shame; so that we would no longer have sickness; and so that we would no longer be without hope. The Messiah is now seated at the right hand of God, in God's presence always interceding for us. He's 'seated' in the heavenlies, as it says in Ephesians, because His work is completed, finished, done. There is nothing to add to it. There is no pain, no struggle, no worries, no fear that Jesus wasn't confronted with while on earth. He is full of compassion for us because He knows what we can and cannot bear. He wants to bear us up, to carry us on His shoulders, and He wants to heal us. His throne is a throne of grace, not a throne of judgment. A throne of grace to help in our time of need. You need the spirit of God, Jesus the Christ, to see that God is for you. You can't see God in your power or ability.

> 1 John 4:4 (NASB) says, *"You are from God, little chil-
> dren, and have overcome them; because greater is He who
> is in you than he who is in the world."*

Don't let the devil immobilize you with false fear. He will get you to focus on yourself, on your circumstances, on your pain, and your lack. If you look to God, who is faithful, who is merciful, who is rich in lovingkindness unto you, who or what can come against you? No one! The devil is powerless. God is powerful. The devil will get you to focus on your condition instead of God's promises and instead of God's faithfulness. That's the scheme of someone who's not powerful. Don't be afraid! Only trust Jesus, our Messiah, and our Savior, to heal you. Take one step at a time, knowing that He is with you and He will never leave you nor forsake you.

7.

WHO YOU LOOKIN' AT ANYWAY?

I usually have a high tolerance for pain, but I went through some rough situations that I wouldn't wish on anyone. It was scary for me to have the hospital take out about a liter and a half of fluid from my lungs. It was painful getting the PICC line placed in my left arm. It was terrifying during the procedure because the doctor was struggling, and the music was heavy metal. It was even more painful to have my loved ones see me in my condition. I had lost so much weight by the end of the first cycle of chemo and I was helpless to whisk away my gaunt look from their eyes. The daddy they knew, who was so successful, was just a bag of bones. My heavenly Daddy knew what I was going through. And if I was going to get through this, I had to focus on Daddy God's love for me, *not* my love for Him.

It is comforting to know that we don't have a Savior who isn't touched by our pain. We have a friend in Jesus. We don't have to pretend with Jesus. If we're in pain, He's right there with us ready to give the healing we so desperately need. God came down in the form of a man to show man that His compassion was to know and understand the struggles we face, the hurts we have, and to heal them. No one knew what I was going through. My wife had some sense, but when you get right down to it, she didn't know what I was going through. She wasn't in my body experiencing what I went through. And neither do your loved ones know nor do your friends know either. None of them knew what I was experiencing. It could only be Jesus who can know what you are going through. The One who designed the body, who created me in my mom's womb, the One who loved me from a knowing standpoint - He is the only one who could know what I was going through.

Many times, we want others to know. But they really can't. No one is you. No one has your background. No one has your physical make-up. No one has the hurts you've had both physically and emotionally. We want to be careful not to burden those who are caregivers with "feeling" our pain. They can't. Only Jesus understands what you are going through. Put that burden on Jesus. He is a friend who listens, who does not judge, who fully understands. He was denied, betrayed, and beaten for us. Isaiah says He bore our sicknesses and our pains on the cross. He bore them so we wouldn't have to. We draw near to Him because He understands, because He forgave completely, once and for all. We draw near to him because in Him we find grace to help in our time of need. Don't go it alone but don't depend on others, either. Be aware of Jesus' presence specifically for you. Be aware of His love and care specifically for you. Know in your heart that He delights to be with you.

At some point, I was in a stable enough condition for the doctors and nurses to begin a heavier dosage of chemo. However, I didn't take it very well. I'm not sure if it was the presence of a bedpan on my lap or simply good timing but I emptied whatever I had in my stomach into that bedpan. I hated the violent lurching of vomiting. I vowed not to go through that again by severely limiting my intake of food for the rest of that first cycle of chemo. Ultimately, it meant I would end up weighing about 135-138 pounds at my lowest point; about 70-75 pounds less than what I weigh today! I'm tall,

6'3," and with a slender build. Losing 75 pounds made me look like death. After cleaning me up, the nurse disposed of the waste in the trashcan in the room. This tall grey trashcan, at some point, came to symbolize in my mind all that was trash in my life.

I had lots of time to think because I didn't watch TV. There was nothing good on TV and they only painted pictures of what went wrong or what could go wrong. I didn't want to carry around this mindset. My imagination supplied what TV could not. I was determined to "look at" Christ. Remembering Numbers 21:8, I wanted to see Jesus and be healed. Numbers 21:8 talks of God telling Moses what to do when the Israelites were in the desert dying of serpent bites. It says, "*Make a fiery serpent, and set it on a pole; and it shall be that everyone who is bitten, when he looks at it, will live.*" Today, this is the universal symbol of the healing arts, a serpent wrapped around a brass pole! But what does that mean? A brass pole signified judgment. And since it was nailed and wrapped around the pole, that serpent wasn't going anywhere. Judgment was wrapped around that pole. But why look at it? To live!

This takes place in the Old Testament. The Old Testament is full of shadows of the Messiah for the people of Israel. A shadow isn't the real thing, but it points to the real thing. God could have picked anything, but He chose this serpent on a pole. Why? He loves Israel. He always has, He always will. He was reminding them of the Messiah to come. He too would be nailed to a pole and all of God's judgment against us would be placed on Him. Seeing that would heal everyone who looked at it. I was "*bitten*" with cancer and I needed to "see" my Savior nailed to a cross taking on my judgment so I could live.

But how do you "see" Jesus in a hospital room? I decided to focus on light. The closest light to me was a diode on a panel at the end of my bed. It was an indicator that would sound an alarm if I fell out of the bed. I stared at that diode. I imagined Jesus looking at me and smiling. A big smile. A smile that said, "I am

so glad to see you." I needed that so much. In those first ten days,
I was dying, and my thoughts kept turning to what I could have
done differently with my life. How I could have spent more time
with my children. Time spent that could have been so much more
meaningful, more personal, and considerate of each member of my
wonderful family. I thought of my sins a lot. I thought of all the
kinds of dumb ass things I had done that didn't honor God and all
kinds of things that ultimately weren't good for me and sometimes
weren't good for others around me. And every time I looked at that
stupid trashcan, I imagined these sins of my past. I relived these
sins. I relived doing things that I was now ashamed of.

Condemnation kills. It doesn't heal. It puts you in the wrong
frame of mind. You are looking at yourself, your actions. You are
not looking at God. It distracted me from looking at Jesus in that
hospital room. I turned from the trashcan back to that diode. Jesus
is again smiling like He's so glad to see me. My condemnation
melted away. For whatever reason, it was just Jesus' face that I
would see until one day I was looking at that stupid trashcan and
thinking of my inglorious past and I see Jesus in front of it. This
time I see him from the waist up. He again is looking at me with
that smile that says I love you so much, it is so good to be with
you, I am so glad to be here with you, I am your friend. But His
back is turned toward me. He's big and He has broad shoulders
and a big back. His face is looking at me, but His back is toward
me. He's in front of the stupid trashcan and I see that His back is
ripped to shreds with open tears, everywhere exposing raw muscle.
But He's still smiling at me. By positioning Himself in front of the
trashcan He's telling me not to look at my sins but to look at Him
and what He did for my healing. He wanted me to see what *He
did* for me on that cross, not what I did in my past. He paid for
my healing. After that episode, I never had any other visions while
in the hospital. That vision was a blessing to me. He took a brutal,
inhumane beating for my healing. Stripes caused by whips with

shards of metal or glass attached to them, designed to rip out flesh and any muscle behind it, all for my healing.

In Isaiah 53:4-5 (CJB: Complete Jewish Bible) we read, *⁴In fact, it was our diseases he bore, our pains from which he suffered; yet we regarded him as punished, stricken and afflicted by God. ⁵But he was wounded because of our crimes, crushed because of our sins; the disciplining that makes us whole fell on him, **and by his bruises we are healed**.*

I'm not sure if it was my imagination or if Jesus appeared to me or if it was the chemo drugs making me hallucinate but I never considered my sins again looking at that trashcan. It is so important to understand that condemnation kills. The very beginning of Romans 8 starts with "*Therefore, there is now no condemnation to those who are in Christ Jesus.*" And the very end of that chapter talks about His love for us, *not our love for him.* His love for you enables you to more than overcome, to be more than a conqueror in all of life's situations.

> Romans 8:37 (NKJV), "*Yet in all these things we are more than conquerors through Him who loved us.*"

When someone loves you, you are naturally drawn to them. You enjoy their presence. It is fun to be around this person. You feel better about yourself. Fix your eyes on the one who loves you. Forget about getting the approval of others who are well-meaning people, especially religious people, or even your loved ones, or any other person's approval for that matter. When you fix your eyes on God, you don't get weary or lose heart in this fight of life.

> Hebrews 12:2-3 (NIV) says *²**Let us fix our eyes on Jesus**, the author and perfecter of our faith, who for **the joy set before him** endured the cross, scorning its shame, and sat down at the right hand of the throne of God.*

[3] ***Consider him*** *who endured such opposition from sinful men, so that you will not grow weary and lose heart. (Bold - my emphasis.)*

Don't let anything get in between you and Jesus and His love for you. Don't let your lack of love for Him or your perceived lack of faith get in the way either. Instead focus on Jesus and His love for you and *His* faith to carry out the promises God has given to you.

8.

THE PRESSURE IS ON HIM, NOT YOU

I didn't want to look at myself in the mirror while I was in the hospital. I knew that I could be easily discouraged if I looked and compared myself to others who were either in the hospital or who came to visit. This is the way it is in life. You are distracted when you compare yourself to others. Instead, look unto Jesus the author and finisher of your faith. He is altogether lovely, and He loves you completely, tenderly, and without reservation. Even when it comes to "faith" people look at themselves and judge that they don't have enough faith. Who are they to judge how much faith is required? Instead, focus on Jesus, His faithfulness to you, and God's faithfulness to His word.

Many religious people point to Luke when the apostles asked the Lord how they could increase their faith. But let's look at this passage carefully and see if it's saying what they think it says.

> Luke 17:5-6 (NIV) *⁵The apostles said to the Lord, "Increase our faith!" ⁶He replied, "If you have faith as small as a mustard seed, you can say to this mulberry tree, 'Be uprooted and planted in the sea,' and it will obey you.*

Now, who said, "increase our faith"? The apostles said this. It wasn't the Lord Jesus saying this. Were the apostles perfect? Of course not. Does the Lord have to respond to their question as truth, or is He more likely to address the real issue? The Lord, who is God's wisdom, didn't respond by saying "This is how you increase your faith." Just because the disciples asked the question "how do we increase our faith?" doesn't make it a truth that faith can be increased. The Lord didn't even bother answering what their human minds came up with.

Instead, the Lord zeroed in on what they needed to zero in on, that is, if you have FAITH as a mustard seed, if you SAY to your problem, if you COMMAND with authority, IT, *your problem*, will obey you. Faith doesn't grow or increase; Jesus never said this. **You simply exercise it.** Faith is a "now" thing, not something you tuck away in your closet. You get it from looking at Jesus. He is the author, the finisher of our faith. Many of us believe that faith is some living growing organism in you. It's not! We've all been given the same measure of faith, so we have what we need. In Romans 12:3 (NASB) it says, *"For through the grace given to me I say to everyone among you not to think more highly of himself than he ought to think; but to think so as to have sound judgment, as God has allotted to each a measure of faith."* When God gives a measure, He isn't cheap. He gave us all we needed. We need to exercise it, to use it, to direct it toward the right object – to God and His Son, Jesus the Messiah. Direct it at the promises of God's word which are all available in Christ Jesus. You trusted God to get born again. What's stopping you now. It's usually unbelief, not a lack of faith. It's unbelief you need to get rid of. Unbelief is trusting the circumstances, the blood count, the X-rays, the doctor's opinion more than the promises of God. Look unto Jesus only, open your mouth and command your problem to leave you.

It's His faithfulness that gives you boldness, not your faith. Ephesians 3:12 (CJB) says, *"In union with him, through his faithful-*

ness, we have boldness and confidence when we approach God." Don't let well-meaning religious people get you to focus on you or your faith. Instead, you focus on Christ, the Messiah and His faith to carry out His promises. For example, people will talk about your need to have "more" faith. Huh?!? Where do they get this notion from? I don't read anywhere in the bible where you are told to get "more" faith. Jesus is the author and finisher of our faith. Our faith alone won't cut it. It boils down to "who you lookin' at anyway."

Here's another verse where people twist things about having 'stronger' faith. Everyone talks about having "strong" faith. Where do they get this notion? *Nothing could be further from the truth.* Read it for yourself. Romans 4:20 (NIV) says, *"yet he did not waver through unbelief regarding the promise of God but was strengthened in his faith and gave glory to God".* So that you're not confused, here's another translation to chew on (same verse): Romans 4:20 (ESV) says, *"No unbelief made him waver concerning the promise of God, but he grew strong in his faith as he gave glory to God".*

In both cases and most translations, we are talking about YOU being strengthened in faith. In the present, now, act of faith. In exercising your faith as Jesus instructed the apostles above, YOU get stronger. When you walk in faith, YOU get stronger. How is this done? If you SAY to your problem, if you have FAITH as a mustard seed, if you COMMAND with authority, IT, *your problem,* will obey you. It's not your faith that gets stronger. YOU DO! Don't waver through unbelief by considering the circumstances. Instead, consider the faithfulness of God, the love of God toward you, and YOU'LL be strengthened in your faith toward Jesus Christ. Faith that says God is faithful, faith that says God loves me. Faith that gives glory to God. Sometimes a different way of looking at this is to use the word trust. Trust God that He loves you, trust God that He is faithful. Trust in God who strengthens you and this trust gives glory to God. It's not your actions that give glory to God, it's the act of trusting Him that gives glory to God. Don't look at yourself or your actions, always look at the Messiah.

Sometimes you'll hear talk about 'levels' of faith. There is no such thing in the bible. It's not in the word of God. Levels are for the religions of man, not for Christianity. You are seated in the heavenlies *now*. There is no higher level to aspire to. You, in your flesh, are growing stronger *now*. You grow strong by practicing the faith you've already received! Who cares if it's the size of a mustard seed? Just open your mouth and practice, practice, practice! Don't wait. Start now!

In the beginning of my stay in the hospital I called cancer dead in my body. I spoke verses of scripture over myself. But I still thought some of it depended on me. The way I said it. What I said. How I said it. I left some of it up to me. It's why I didn't receive my healing in the hospital. Remember, it's God's responsibility to carry out His word and He is faithful to do it! We have nothing to do with the increase which comes from God. We look to God because through His love for us, through this knowledge of His love for us, we not only endure, but we are more than conquerors (Romans 8:37). God is faithful. Hebrews 10:23 (NIV) says: *Let us hold unswervingly to the hope we profess, for he who promised is faithful.* In 2 Thessalonians 3:3 (NIV) we read, *But the Lord is faithful, and he will strengthen and protect you from the evil one.* Don't do the Lord's job. The Lord Jesus has all the faith you need. He will strengthen you. He will establish you. He will heal you. He is the one who protects you from evil.

The old covenant way of "discipline" is focused on you. This is where you can impress others with exploits you've done in the flesh. How long you've prayed, how many verses you've memorized, etc. This leads to comparing you with others because it elevates your life. This is the old way of the law, of prospering under the old covenant. We are no longer under the old covenant. We let God perform. We no longer have to perform to receive. We are not under law but grace.

Let's not confuse God's performance with our faith. Our faith isn't performance. It's simple trust in God. It's trust that His promises are sealed unto us because of the finished work of Jesus Christ. These promises in the new covenant are FOR YOU. When you trust God, you are allowing the grace of our Lord Jesus Christ to work in you. Faith rests on grace, on His grace, and not on your works. That's why in Romans 4:16 (ESV) it says, *That is why it depends on faith, so that the promise may rest on grace and be guaranteed to all his offspring—not only to the adherent of the law but also to the one who shares the faith of Abraham, who is the father of us all.*

Let's not complicate faith. When you believe, you speak out loud His promises. You command your problems, and they obey you. And then you take one step at a time based on the promise of God. One step at a time, that's all it takes. Don't focus on tomorrow, or one hour from now. Just believe right now and act in the now of faith.

9.

THE FATHER'S LOVE FOR YOU

When Jesus was on earth, He taught people what God's love looks like. An example of this love can be found in the parable of The Prodigal Son, a misnomer of a title. This is not a parable about the son, but about our Father, God. It's about the Father's love for us. I want and need you to understand how much God loves you. It's not like man's love for his fellow man. It's God-love, for you. Having gone through all that I went through, I hung unto the truth that Jesus loves me, and it was more than a love thought for Him. It was a love that was real. It was His love that understood me. It was His love that knew my frame, how I deal with situations, and that knew what was best for me. The parable of The Prodigal Son shows God's heart of love *for you*. Read this story for the first time with different eyes. Remember, you are more than a conqueror through HIS love for you (Romans 8:37).

> Luke 15:11-32 (NIV) reads *11 Jesus continued: "There was a man who had two sons. 12 The younger one said to his father, 'Father, give me my share of the estate.' So, he divided his property between them. 13 "Not long after that, the younger son got together all he had, set off for a distant*

country and there squandered his wealth in wild living.
¹⁴After he had spent everything, there was a severe famine
in that whole country, and he began to be in need. ¹⁵So
he went and hired himself out to a citizen of that country,
who sent him to his fields to feed pigs. ¹⁶He longed to fill
his stomach with the pods that the pigs were eating, but
no one gave him anything. ¹⁷"When he came to his senses,
he said, 'How many of my father's hired men have food
to spare, and here I am starving to death! ¹⁸I will set out
and go back to my father and say to him: Father, I have
sinned against heaven and against you. ¹⁹I am no longer
worthy to be called your son; make me like one of your
hired men.' ²⁰So he got up and went to his father. "But
while he was still a long way off, his father saw him and
was filled with compassion for him; he ran to his son,
threw his arms around him and kissed him. ²¹"The son
said to him, 'Father, I have sinned against heaven and
against you. I am no longer worthy to be called your son.'
²²"But the father said to his servants, 'Quick! Bring the
best robe and put it on him. Put a ring on his finger and
sandals on his feet. ²³Bring the fattened calf and kill it.
Let's have a feast and celebrate. ²⁴For this son of mine was
dead and is alive again; he was lost and is found.' So, they
began to celebrate. ²⁵"Meanwhile, the older son was in the
field. When he came near the house, he heard music and
dancing. ²⁶So he called one of the servants and asked him
what was going on. ²⁷'Your brother has come,' he replied,
'and your father has killed the fattened calf because he has
him back safe and sound.' ²⁸"The older brother became
angry and refused to go in. So, his father went out and
pleaded with him. ²⁹But he answered his father, 'Look! All
these years I've been slaving for you and never disobeyed
your orders. Yet you never gave me even a young goat so

I could celebrate with my friends. [30]*But when this son of yours who has squandered your property with prostitutes comes home, you kill the fattened calf for him!'* [31]*"'My son,' the father said, 'you are always with me, and everything I have is yours.* [32]*But we had to celebrate and be glad, because this brother of yours was dead and is alive again; he was lost and is found.'"*

Under the old covenant of the law, we were commanded to love God. It's a standard we couldn't and can't live up to. We aren't God. It was held up as part of the law in Deuteronomy 6:4-5. The law was designed to bring us to Christ, the Messiah, because we needed to know and understand that we can't be good enough on our terms. In this New Covenant that we live in, because of Christ, our Messiah, we focus on His love for us, not our love for Him.

He is the one who loves us with all His heart, His soul, His mind, His strength! Just like the Apostle John, who considered himself the apostle whom Jesus loved, so you should consider yourself the man or woman that Jesus loves. Get a laser-like focus on Jesus' love for you. Call yourself the disciple whom Jesus loves. It's not being arrogant. It's true! No matter what you do or what you have done or what you are currently experiencing, His love for you is unconditional, never-changing and never-condemning. Identify with His love for you and you will more than overcome in every situation life presents to you. It's the promise of Romans 8:37 realized in our Messiah. It's how you're going to receive your healing from Jesus Christ.

Another point I want you to take away from this parable is this: God has never been in a hurry for anything in the Old Testament. But He's now in a hurry for you! Why? Because He loves you. Let's look at verse 20.

"So, he got up and went to his father. "But while he was

still a long way off, his father saw him and was filled with compassion for him; he ran to his son, threw his arms around him and kissed him."

The son, who was astray, got up and went to visit his father. But while he was still a long way off, **the father *ran* to meet him**. Sometimes you'll hear religious people use phrases like "we need to be running to God" and similar statements. *This is a story of when God ran. And He ran for us*. It's so urgent for Him to fellowship with you, to see you, to love you, that He runs to you. He loves you so much. God isn't running because He's angry. In verse 20, the father, who is a type for our heavenly Father, is filled with compassion. God is filled with compassion for you! Can you imagine how big God is? Don't try - it might hurt your head. This big God is a Father who's filled with a flood of compassion *for you*. This isn't a trickle of compassion either. It's for us. And when He reaches you, He does things that embarrass you, like kissing you when He sees you. He loves you so much that He wants to show it to you.

Now look at the next verse. *"The son said to him, 'Father, I have sinned against heaven and against you. I am no longer worthy to be called your son.'* The son has this rehearsed line of contrition. It's bogus. It's talking about being a slave so he can fill his stomach again with decent food. It's bargaining with God. It's acting like you're a hired servant. This is the way of religion. Religion is for beggars. This son didn't know His Father's heart. This son thought, if I do something for you, you'll give me servant's crumbs. But to God, you are not a hired servant. **You are the love of His life.** He loves you. Immediately the father cuts off the son from this rehearsed old covenant slave talk of serving God. He won't hear another word of this religious drivel coming from his son. *"But the father said to his servants, 'Quick! Bring the best robe and put it on him. Put a ring on his finger and sandals on his feet.* ²³*Bring the fattened calf and kill it. Let's have a feast and celebrate.*

Jesus is the Lord our Righteousness and we have received from Him the gift of righteousness or rightness with God. We are clothed with His robe of righteousness, not just any robe, but the best robe there is! Let's celebrate! This is God's heart of love for you. It is all wrapped up in this gift He gave you: His Son, Jesus Christ.

How does the other son react? Like a typical religious servant-type person would. He gets angry if he isn't compensated for his good works. The father goes out to meet with the angry son and pleads with him. But the son doesn't want anything to do with the father. He instead points to himself. What happens when you take your eyes off God? You naturally put the spotlight on you. He points to himself by comparing himself with his brother. *The more religious you are, the more you compare yourself with others.* "This son of yours" sinned, the scorned brother says, and "you give him the fatted calf." What does God then remind him of? *"'My son,' the father said, 'you are always with me, and everything I have is yours.*

You see, the son felt he had to work for God's blessings. But everything God has was the son's and it was for the son's *taking*. But the dutiful son wanted to earn it. He wanted it owed to him because of his good works, his work for his father. That's religious stinkin' thinkin'. That's what I had early in my hospital stay when I tried to bargain my way to healing. That's not the father's thinking and it's not our heavenly Father's thinking either. "***Everything I have is yours.***" Does He have peace? Yes. Does He have abundance and lacks nothing? Yes. Does He have good health? Yes. Everything I have is yours for the taking. Take it.

Love is given so that it can be received. But the dutiful son wanted to earn it. We don't want to know God like this. We think we do but it's from an old covenant mindset if we think like the angry son who wanted to earn blessings, or like the prodigal son, who wanted to act like a hired servant and earn the crumbs of a hired servant. Jesus said on the cross "*It is finished!*" There isn't anything left for us to do except to learn how to receive His love and the blessings He purchased for us with His sacrifice on the cross. This is not a prosperity gospel or how to amass things for yourself. This is how to receive what you need from a God who loves you so intensely that He runs to you. The prodigal son wasted everything the father gave him. Did that stop the father from giving him more? A thousand times no! God is more than wanting to always supply all your need according to His riches in Christ Jesus no matter what you've done in your past. Philippians 4:19 (NASB) says, *And my God will supply all your needs according to His riches in glory in Christ Jesus.* You don't earn His blessings for you.

There is no fear in love, but perfect love casts out fear. It's not your love for God that casts out fear as the religious of our day would like you to believe, rather, it's His love for you that casts out fear. The place where there is no fear is in His love for you. Fear has to do with punishment because you haven't performed well enough. God isn't looking for you to perform. He wants you to receive His love for you! Don't be afraid. Instead, be filled with His love for you.

Christ said in John 14:27 (NIV), *Peace I leave with you; my peace I give you. I do not give to you as the world gives. Do not let your hearts be troubled and do not be afraid.* Jesus doesn't give like the world gives. This peace is Shalom. John 14:27 (CJB) says "What I am leaving with you is shalom—I am giving you my shalom. I don't give the way the world gives. Don't let yourselves be upset or frightened." Jews understand this. Shalom isn't just the absence of conflict, it's the absence of stress and the absence of strife. When you are satisfied or "full" in your life, there is no lack, no worry, and no stress. Life is rich and good and full of blessings, full of Shalom. If Jesus is giving us His Shalom then let's take it. You take it when you are not afraid or troubled. You are not afraid or troubled when you know and believe God's love for you.

Religious people get you to focus on your love for Him. And religious people always talk about what they're doing for God. They say silly things like "running to Jesus" or they sing silly songs like 'I will always love you Jesus'. What a bunch of phooey! *I will never always love Jesus.* Man, I want to, but I know I won't. You read that right, in black and white. I will in heaven, but in this fleshly body on earth, I won't always love Him. Let's get honest here. Instead, I'll praise God for His love for me, how it knows no end, how it uplifts me, how it is unique for me! Why do you think most Christians die, divorce, and just struggle at rates equal to and usually greater than society in general? It's because we don't know the God of the New Covenant; we only know the laws of the Old Covenant that are impossible for us to live up to. The laws were meant to drive us to our need for a Messiah because we can't uphold the laws, not in their entirety and not in the sense that a perfect God thinks of.

The God many religious institutions know is a distant, legalistic God. A God that is called Mighty, Almighty, and other great names but never as our Father, as Jesus referred to Him and never as our Daddy, or Abba, as the apostle Paul revealed in the book of Romans. Jesus was the first to call God His heavenly Father. He's tipping us off to something in the relationship we should look for with God. In the New Covenant we go further than ever before in our relationship with God. We have such a loving God that in the book of Romans we are told we are to call God, Daddy, or "Abba" Father. It's a term of endearment that's like Poppa, or Dada, or what we would call Daddy. He's our heavenly Daddy! Romans 8:15 (NASB) says, *For you have not received a spirit of slavery leading to fear again, but you have received a spirit of adoption as sons by which we cry out, "Abba! Father!"*

Don't listen to voices that portray God as a distant God. We should know God intimately as our Daddy. There's a difference between knowing God and knowing things about Him. Knowing God implies a relationship, and we have this relationship because of Jesus, not because of any good we do.

Jesus loves you so much He isn't concerned with your outward appearance. He isn't concerned with what laws you've kept. He isn't concerned with you looking or acting like everyone else. Sometimes we are taught to act nice, to play nice, and to just be nice. "Be like Jesus", they'll say. Instead, you should be *looking at* Jesus, the author and finisher of your faith, looking at *His love for you*, His desire to bless you with His Shalom or peace and just be yourself. He loves you. Don't ever stray from this. Shout it out! Jesus loves you with all His heart, His soul, His mind, and His strength. He loves you! You draw near to God with confidence when you know this.

10.

BECOME JESUS CONSCIOUS

One night during the first week to ten days of being in the Intensive Care Unit, I was soundly asleep at about 2 a.m. when I suddenly heard a bang! I woke up startled, nurses burst into my room, all the lights were turned on, commands were being shouted. Nurses and orderlies, perhaps five or six of them, furiously went about the room and seemed bent on a mission. I felt like I was on a movie set and I was going through an emergency scene. Nurses were removing the EKG stuff stuck to my chest and arms. Other nurses were running around getting my belongings! Where am I going? What's happening to me? Why is everyone in such a hurry? One of the nurses explained to me that someone needed the room more than I did. In a matter of four to five minutes, I was loaded into a wheelchair with an IV by my side while they wheeled me off to another room on another floor. That room became my home for the next several weeks.

There were multiple other times when things needed to happen quickly. When I first went to the emergency room and was misdiagnosed with an ulcer, I was in pain and needed quick relief. Later the next morning, I needed to get out of that hospital, and I put on my best game face that everything was fine so I could leave quickly.

Six weeks later, when the diagnosis of cancer was confirmed, I couldn't make it to the emergency room on my own and the doctors insisted I be taken by ambulance. I seemed to always be in a hurry. But in between these urgencies, my wife and I tried to have some semblance of normalcy. Sometimes she would stay through the night and sometimes it was easier for Penny to spend that time with my daughter Alyson who had come from Austin to be with her.

Many times in that hospital room I did things that were not godly. Sometimes I was afraid[5], sometimes I didn't believe[6], sometimes I thought ill of others. There were many times that I would be arguing with my wife. Sometimes it was so bad between my wife and I that she didn't want to sleep in the hospital room with me on those nights. I can be a jerk at times. But this didn't disqualify me from receiving my healing. Your sins won't stop God from healing you. Your sins are not more powerful than God's finished work on the cross. You need to get to the place where you are only conscious of your loving Savior loving you. You are only conscious of His healing for you. You are only conscious of His peace, shalom, for you. You are forgiven. Completely. This is the right relationship you have with God because of the Messiah, not because of your good works and not because of your bad sins[7].

I need you to be Jesus conscious or Son conscious so you can take what's rightfully yours in Christ. The sooner you believe in the righteousness God gave you through Christ, the quicker you

---

[5] 2 Timothy 1:7 (NKJV) For God has not given us a spirit of fear, but of power and of love and of a sound mind.

[6] Romans 14:23 (NIV) But the man who has doubts is condemned if he eats, because his eating is not from faith; and everything that does not come from faith is sin.

[7] I'm not advocating that people sin or that it's even ok to sin. I just know that I sin every day and I'm not going to let that define my relationship with God. Jesus is going to define my relationship with God.

can be healed. Righteousness is your rightness before God. This rightness is not dependent on you. That means it's not dependent on your sins either - it's not dependent on yesterday's sins, today's sins, or tomorrow's sins. You are right with God because of the "finished" work of Jesus on the cross. That's why we look at the cross. It's over. It's paid for. There is nothing more you can do to be right with God. He made you right with Him. ***You had nothing to do with it.*** When Jesus gave up His spirit, He said "*It is finished!*" He didn't say, "I need you guys and gals to take over from here. I need you to pick up where I left off." Jesus isn't an example of how to be a good person either. Instead, Jesus is our Savior. He is more than an example. He is our Shepherd, the Lord our Righteousness, our Healer, and our Deliverer. The Messiah became a man so He could identify with our pains and sorrows. He was crucified so we wouldn't have to continue with pains and sorrows.

In John 10:7, it says that Jesus is the door **of** the sheep. He's not the door **to** the sheep. ***He is the door.*** You are not going to enter healing except through Jesus. You aren't going to enter the room of peace except through the door of Jesus. Don't get tricked into looking at how you can "improve" yourself. Religious people don't point to Jesus, they point to themselves and get you to focus on improving yourself. I can't improve on what Jesus did on the cross so why do I need to worry about improving myself.

You know, when I'm in the presence of someone who loves me, I am enthralled with their love. I'm a better person. This is what marriage is like. In my best moments with my wife, I am so loved by her and so blessed to be with her, face to face. Loving her and being loved by her. In your lover's arms and eyes, you are a better person! That's what it is like to be with Jesus in His presence. The righteous man or woman, that's you or me if you are born again, are only required to live by faith. Think of faith, not as a list of do's and don'ts to agree with, but as a now-trust in what God has written in the word of God, and specifically written in the church

epistles that apply to you. These are now-promises from God to
you. Trust His word. Trust His Son, the word made flesh. Trust
the promises of God in His love letters of the epistles to the saints,
Romans through Thessalonians.

You see, to be born again is quite simple. You simply confess
with your mouth that Jesus is Lord and believe in your heart that
God raised Him from the dead. We don't need to confess our sins.
Why? Because there is only one verse in the new covenant that talks
about this and it would take another book to explain why that one
verse is misunderstood. God has, because of all judgment being
placed on Jesus on the cross, forgiven us for all sins. And He says
<u>He remembers</u> them NO MORE[8]. They are not in His memory

---

[8] Hebrews 10:15-23 (NIV) [15]The Holy Spirit also testifies to us about this.
First, he says: [16]"This is the covenant I will make with them after that time,
says the Lord. I will put my laws in their hearts, and I will write them on their
minds." [17]Then he adds: **"Their sins and lawless acts I will remember no
more."** [18]And where these have been forgiven, there is no longer any sacrifice
for sin. [19]Therefore, brothers, since we have confidence to enter the Most Holy
Place by the blood of Jesus, [20]by a new and living way opened for us through
the curtain, that is, his body, [21]and since we have a great priest over the house
of God, [22]let us draw near to God with a sincere heart in full assurance of faith,
having our hearts sprinkled to cleanse us from a guilty conscience and having
our bodies washed with pure water. [23]Let us hold unswervingly to the hope we
profess, for he who promised is faithful.

This is taken from the Old Testament verses in Jeremiah.

Jeremiah 31:31-34 (NIV) [31]"The time is coming," declares the LORD, "when I
will make a new covenant with the house of Israel and with the house of Judah.
[32]It will not be like the covenant I made with their forefathers when I took
them by the hand to lead them out of Egypt, because they broke my covenant,
though I was a husband to them," declares the LORD. [33]"This is the covenant
I will make with the house of Israel after that time," declares the LORD. "I will
put my law in their minds and write it on their hearts. I will be their God, and
they will be my people. [34]No longer will a man teach his neighbor, or a man

or His thinking. If He doesn't remember them, why do we want to remember them? You are no longer condemned by God. Jesus took our full punishment upon Him. There is no punishment from God left for us. God has identified you with His Son, Jesus.

Look at what Hebrews 10:1-4 says to us in the Complete Jewish Bible (CJB), *¹For the Torah has in it a shadow of the good things to come, but not the actual manifestation of the originals. Therefore, it can never, by means of the same sacrifices repeated endlessly year after year, bring to the goal those who approach the Holy Place to offer them. ²Otherwise, wouldn't the offering of those sacrifices have ceased?* **For if the people performing the service had been cleansed once and for all, they would no longer have sins on their conscience.** *³No, it is quite the contrary—in these sacrifices is a reminder of sins, year after year. ⁴For it is impossible that the blood of bulls and goats should take away sins.*

We have been cleaned once and for all and **we should no longer have sins on our conscience.** The day of atonement was a shadow of what we have every day, not just once a year - complete and utter atonement, once and for all, made by our Savior Jesus, on the cross. This means that we should *"no longer have sins on our conscience."* So instead of being *sin conscious* we need to be *Son conscious.* My righteousness, a gift from God, doesn't go away if I sin.

---

his brother, saying, 'Know the LORD,' because they will all know me, from the least of them to the greatest," declares the LORD. **"For I will forgive their wickedness and will remember their sins no more."**

11.

WHAT DO YOU "DO" TO RECEIVE HEALING?

I'd just had a doctor visit at my bedside, one of many which would take place in a regular cadence. With the doctor now gone, my room was quiet and peaceful again. No one was bothering me. I shifted myself with some effort to move into a more comfortable position, slightly elevated, pillows under my left arm, staring down at my swollen legs. What do I do? What can I do? I resigned myself to the fact that I was helpless. I couldn't do a thing. I was focused on talking with God now and I told my heavenly Daddy, *"God, I can't do anything for myself lying here, but I can praise you and I can thank you for all the good you have done for me and all the good you are in my life."* I then softly spoke in tongues, knowing I was praising God, uttering perfect praises to Him (Acts 10:46). Sometimes you just don't know what to say or what to pray. In those situations, it's better just to praise God. Tell God how wonderful He is. Tell God how thankful you are for His Son Jesus having paid for every sin, for every healing, for every shame, for your peace that goes beyond your understanding. You don't have to jump around and shout out loud. You have a unique personality. Be yourself. Be who God made you. Praise God the way you would praise someone but with a level of thanks that wells up from within your heart. After a few minutes, I drifted off to sleep.

When I started to get better, I read. I didn't read my bible because most of my life was spent studying the word and so I tend to study when I read the word. Studying for me is finding out what was said and why it was said. In other words, what does this word mean? What is God saying here? Things like that. My daughter Alyson had brought me a book from home that I had bought and wanted to read but hadn't quite gotten around to it. It was a book by Pastor Joseph Prince called "*The Power of Right Believing.*" What I remember most about the book was the power of worship and how David worshipped with his men in the cave of Adullam, 300 of them, at perhaps what looked like one of the lowest points in David's life. Psalm 34 was written during this incredibly low time in David's life. As Pastor Joseph Prince said in this book, "*As we worship Him and become utterly lost in His magnificent love for us, something happens to us. We are forever changed and transformed in His presence. All fears, worries, and anxieties depart when Jesus is exalted in our worship.*"[9] There is healing in worship! Here's what David wrote in Psalm 34:

> Psalms 34:1-4 (NASB) [1]I will bless the LORD at all times; His praise shall continually be in my mouth. [2]My soul will make its boast in the LORD; The humble will hear it and rejoice. [3]O magnify the LORD with me and let us exalt His name together. [4]I sought the LORD, and He answered me, and delivered me from all my fears.

[9] Excerpt From: Joseph Prince. "The Power of Right Believing." iBooks. https://itunes.apple.com/us/book/the-power-of-right-believing/id645584866?mt=11

I highly recommend Pastor Joseph Prince's book and all the books written by Pastor Joseph Prince. I believe when I let go of my situation and began worshipping the Lord that my situation turned for the better. Let go of yourself and let God be God. He is your strength, and He is your healer!

It's quite common for religious people to console people who are sick with the baloney that being sick is good for them. It was good for Paul so you can suck it up is how this line of religious stinkin' thinkin' works. A lot of times they point to Paul's thorn in the flesh. Here's the verse in question: 2 Corinthians 12:7 (NASB) says, *Because of the surpassing greatness of the revelations, for this reason, to keep me from exalting myself, there was given me a thorn in the flesh, a messenger of Satan to torment me—to keep me from exalting myself! [8] Concerning this I implored the Lord three times that it might leave me. [9] And He has said to me, "My grace is sufficient for you, for power is perfected in weakness." Most gladly, therefore, I will rather boast about my weaknesses, so that the power of Christ may dwell in me.*

Well, let's look at these verses in a bit more detail. A thorn in the flesh, according to the first occurrence of the word in the Old Testament, is someone who is a pain in the ass. This is how we would say thorn in our common vernacular. It's not an actual thorn in your side. It's a person, not a sickness. Here's the first occurrence in the OT: Numbers 33:55 (NASB) reads, *But if you do not drive out the inhabitants of the land from before you, then it shall come about that those whom you let remain of them will become as pricks in your eyes and as thorns in your sides, and they will trouble you in the land in which you live.*

Let's go back to what Paul was talking about because this is important to you in the suffering you may now be experiencing. Note verse 7 in 2 Corinthians 12 above - the thorn was a messenger of Satan. This person bothering Paul, probably drawing attention to him or herself, was not walking by the spirit of God but by the prince of the darkness of the air. This person's actions were meant to trouble Paul. This is what a pain in the ass does. Three times Paul asked Jesus to take it from him. Jesus told Paul His grace was sufficient for Paul. Paul heard the words and concluded that Christ's power was perfected or completed in weakness. **Here we're talking about Paul's weakness to deal with the situation. We are not talking about any sickness in his flesh**. Then Paul says "*Most gladly*" I'll boast in my weaknesses so that the power of Christ would dwell in me.

Now think about this. You can rejoice in whatever situation you are in. It doesn't say to rejoice FOR every situation you are in, like an illness, or that you are suffering in some way. That would be insanity. God didn't design our bodies to like or want sickness and disease and He didn't design our bodies to need sickness or disease or stress. But because many religious people don't know how to explain this from the word of God, they punt. When you are weak, when you don't have the strength to move on, that's when you rejoice in the Lord. Why? Because **He is our strength. His power** is "perfected" or "completed" in our weakness. **It's all about Him, and not about you.**

God's power isn't as awe-inspiring when we can do the job ourselves. Who needs God in situations where you can handle it? You see, He gets the glory when you can't get it done with your efforts and your power. Simple enough, huh? Not really. We are trained since birth to trust the things we can see and touch. To trust God, we must move away from what our senses tell us and focus on what the word of God tells us. We look unto the Messiah, the author, and finisher of our faith. Christ is the Word made flesh. When we look at Him and focus on who He is, and what He's "finished" for us, the world around us falls away. We can't do anything good for ourselves, we can't heal ourselves, we can't even bring ourselves real peace, but God can, and He's already demonstrated this when He came to the earth in the form of a man.

After the first 10-14 days, my wife and I began to put together a list of what we would do once I got out. It helped to keep my mind off the current circumstances and focus on something else. I believe this was a blessing to my wife as well because we could change what we were preoccupied with. This wasn't a "bucket list" of what I wanted to do before I died. It was just a list of things Penny and I wanted to enjoy doing together after I was healed. It included things like going to the UK on a Rick Steve's Tour, visiting the Grand Canyon (done in 2017), going to Singapore to see Pastor Joseph Prince preach (done in September/October 2018), and so on. This helped Penny as a caregiver to take her focus off the daily stats the doctors were giving her (blood cell counts and other things). It helped both of us to relax. Rest is important. Think of rest as the absence of stress, not simply being still.

It doesn't mean you don't do anything, but what you do is **rest in what He can do**. You work knowing that it is not your work getting you to where you are going in life but His work in you. His work will deliver your victory. What is your trust in? In what you can see or feel with your senses or in what God's word says? Maybe you have to take a pill ordered by the doctor. So what! Remember, there is no condemnation in Christ. Take the pill but trust in God. When you take that pill or pills just simply say, "I cannot heal myself Lord, but you can heal me. I am trusting you, Lord." Let God work in you. Don't let your circumstances get in the way or cloud your judgment. He is at work within you to will and to work for His good pleasure.

Don't confuse your circumstance with His will. His will is only good for you. His will is healing to your life. In heaven, there are only healed people. We pray for His will to be done on earth *as it is in heaven*. Trust Him to carry out His good will. When He was on earth, He healed everyone that came to Him for healing. Would God do any less for us today? We've all heard the phrase, Jesus is the same yesterday, today and forever (it's in the bible[10]). Does Jesus now not heal? Has He changed? Is that the way The Messiah would be? NO! His will is accomplished by God Himself, by His strength and not by your efforts or by your strength. Rest and receive your healing. Rest in your weakness in the flesh. Another way to put this: rest in your inability to heal yourself. When you are weak, He is strong. Just rest in your weakness in the flesh and rest in His ability in the Spirit.

Sickness is an enemy, but you can't fight it. Early on I tried fighting cancer. I felt like I was fighting for my life. And sometimes the onslaught seemed relentless. It was as if some force were trying to see just how much I could take. But I learned that I couldn't fight cancer on my own. Instead, I decided to let the Lord do the fighting. I had given up and instead praised God for His goodness, not for this sickness! That's rejoicing in your weakness. In Ephesians, we are described as seated in the heavenlies in Christ. If Christ is **seated** at the right hand of the Father, then He is at a position of rest. If we're seated with Him, then we're in the same position of rest. He's at rest because His work is finished. We're at rest because His work is finished. We are in Him and we are at rest.

How does God see you? He sees you as perfect *and* He sees you healed. You see, you had nothing to do with your perfection, except to believe in the Messiah's finished work. He made you perfect. Perhaps the outside man hasn't caught up with the spiritual reality, but it will. In Hebrews 10:12-18 (NASB) we have: *[12] but He, having offered **one sacrifice for sins for all time**, SAT DOWN AT THE RIGHT HAND OF GOD, [13] waiting from that time onward UNTIL HIS ENEMIES BE MADE A FOOTSTOOL FOR HIS FEET. [14] For **by one offering He has perfected for all time those who are sanctified**. [15] And the Holy Spirit also testifies to us; for after saying, [16] "THIS IS THE COVENANT THAT **I WILL***

---

[10] Hebrews 13:8 (NASB) Jesus Christ *is* the same yesterday and today and forever.

*MAKE WITH THEM AFTER THOSE DAYS, SAYS THE LORD: **I WILL** PUT MY LAWS UPON THEIR HEART, AND ON THEIR MIND **I WILL** WRITE THEM," He then says, [17] "AND THEIR SINS AND THEIR LAWLESS DEEDS **I WILL** REMEMBER NO MORE." [18] Now **where there is forgiveness of these things, there is no longer any offering for sin.***

Please note: the ALL CAPS are not God shouting at us but it's a way the translators show that this is a reference or a quote from the Old Testament. It shows that this was a promise in the Old Testament meant for us today. We are sanctified or set apart and perfected, *past tense*: we were made perfect, in one single action - the finished work of our Messiah on the cross! God sees you as perfect. Rejoice in that perfection no matter what the circumstances!

Hebrews 4:10 (NASB) says, *"For the one who has entered His rest has himself also rested from his works, as God did from His."* Why do this? In order that you won't fall. When you are at rest in Christ, the Messiah, you aren't struggling. You aren't stressed. You aren't disobeying. This may sound crazy to you but to be in a state of unrest is disobeying God. Why? Because you're not trusting that He has your back. You're not trusting that what He said was true. The very next verse in Hebrews 4:11 (NASB) says, *"Therefore let us be diligent to enter that rest, so that no one will fall, through following the same example of disobedience."*

To receive from God, be at rest. Trust God. One moment at a time. Let your Daddy God take care of you. Just let go and let Him be God for you. What was the example that God was talking about in Hebrews 4:11? It was not entering the Promised Land because they thought the giants were too big for them. Well, of course, the giants were too big for THEM, but they were not too big for GOD. The Promised Land for us today is the land purchased by the blood of Jesus Christ. The land of milk and honey where God cares for your every need, big or small. Where the grapes that you didn't plant are too large for you, where the homes weren't built by you, where the prosperity did not come by your hand.

The only work we have in this life is to enter His rest now. Why does God consider that work? Because it's the most challenging thing you'll ever face as a believer. It is completely counter to your flesh way of thinking. It is one moment at a time. You can't store it up to use it tomorrow. It's NOW. To rest in God's love for you knowing that He provides for you and will provide for you, that He is your peace, your justifier, your healer, your strength requires diligence. Sometimes it feels like a 24/7 thing, especially when you are near death with cancer. But it's the same for all walks in this life. Even though you may "work" a job or "work" as a parent/teacher/husband/wife/etc., your real "work" is not to trust your work as your deliverer but to trust the Lord our Righteousness as your deliverer. This 'entering in' requires diligence on our part. This isn't like a vacation. It's more like a kind of mindfulness that God is always providing for you now. Right now. Trust God. Trust His promises for you. Trust that you can let go of any cares you have and focus on the task at hand even when that task is to just listen. This is the mindfulness the world wants but doesn't understand. It's a mindfulness that God is with you providing for you right now at this moment. You can let go and let God be your provider, your rock, your fortress, your deliverer, and your strength when you can't go on by yourself. Let God be God for you.

Don't Fight Cancer! It's Not Your Battle.

It's not our fight. It's His. It's not our battle. It's His. If we make it our fight, why should God work? We get all the glory. This runs counterintuitive to how we've been brought up. "God helps those who help themselves" is NOT in your bible. His power is made perfect in your weakness, in your "I can't do this", in your "I need you", in your "I need your wisdom because I don't know what to do", in your "I need your favor God because I don't see how this can be done", in your "I need your healing God because I can't heal myself." Jesus did all the work for you at the cross. He paid a very real price. Everything that happened at the cross was done so that everything He has would be yours. He took on your shame, your judgment, your sickness and disease, and your sin so that you would receive His righteousness, His lack of shame, His health, and His peace. In other words, so that you would *reign in life*, not just "survive." I'm not a cancer survivor, I'm a reign-in-lifer! The only thing you need to do is to rest in *His* finished work. Just cease from your efforts and let Him heal you. I believe this "letting go" let me receive from God. I didn't know what to "do", but I knew if I just let go and let God, that He would deliver me. I just didn't understand how it would be done.

> In Matthew 11:28-30 (NASB) Jesus says, [28]*"Come to Me, all who are weary and heavy-laden, and I will give you rest.* [29]*"Take My yoke upon you and learn from Me, for I am gentle and humble in heart, and YOU WILL FIND REST FOR YOUR SOULS.* [30]*"For My yoke is easy and My burden is light."*

He gives us rest and it is rest for our souls, not our bodies. Sickness in your flesh is a body that's not at rest. It's fighting for life. Before your body heals, let your soul receive *His* rest. Sickness in your mind is a soul that's not in rest. Your soul is what makes you unique. It is not your spirit which is from God. Your soul is not the spirit of Jesus Christ. Instead, your soul is made up of your mind, your will, and your emotions. Think of your soul as the DNA God gave you. Your mind finds rest in Christ, your will finds rest in Christ, and your emotions find rest in Christ. And Jesus asks us to "take" it from Him. Don't wait for it to drop in your lap. Take it! Take it by now-faith, by now-trust. Everything for the child of God is received by trusting God or by faith. When you are at the feet of Jesus, you get to "*learn from*" Him. As a teacher, He's gentle and humble in heart. He's not condemning, He's not going to trick you with a 'gotcha' as I know some religious folks have done to me. He loves you with gentleness and humbleness of heart. Whether your sickness is in your flesh, like with cancer, or in your mind, like with depression, let Him heal you. Remember, there is no condemnation in Christ whether you are sick in your flesh or sick in your mind. Take and receive the good God has for you.

Jesus, our Messiah, said, "*come to me.*" We are not to ask Christ to come to us but rather He asks us to go to Him. And when we do, He gives the rest. When we are diligent or as the King James Version says when we "labor" to enter His rest, we are diligent to receive from Him! Look at 3 John 2 (ESV) which reads, *Beloved, I pray that all may go well with you and that you may be in good health,* ***as it goes well with your soul.*** You see, you need to be at rest in your soul for your body to heal. You need to be free from stress in your mind, from stress in your will, and stress in your emotions. As it goes well with your soul, so may you be in good health!

What do you "do" while you're waiting, and I would say, hoping on the Lord? I tried listening to a friend's list of music. It was okay. The words in the songs were words of encouragement but they didn't do anything for me. Instead, I would just rest. I would sit there in bed and just think. But mostly I would praise God and have thankful thoughts for His Son, Jesus, and what He meant to my life. Thanking God is a simple but effective thing for you to do when you don't know what else to do. For your sake, don't worry, don't fear, and don't mumble your problems to anyone or even to yourself out loud.

In Joshua 1:8-9 (ESV), we read: [8]"This Book of the Law shall not depart from your mouth, but you shall meditate on it day and night, so that you may be careful to do according to all that is written in it. For then you will make your way prosperous, and then you will have good success. ⁹Have I not commanded you? Be strong and courageous. Do not be frightened, and do not be dismayed, for the LORD your God is with you wherever you go."

Success does not mean meditating in a lotus position like I used to do early in my life. When God says something in His word, it's important to understand what He is talking about, not what you're thinking about. The word for 'meditate' in Joshua 1:8 is the Hebrew word 'hagah,' which means to mutter, to utter, or to make a sound, etc. Basically, it's mumbling out loud! What do most people mumble or mutter aloud about? Their problems! "The economy is going downhill," "jobs aren't as plentiful as they used to be," "I never really get a break," and on and on and on. Don't do this. Instead, speak God's word out loud. God knows people like to mutter out loud and so He made it easy for us to be successful doing what we're inclined to do naturally anyway. But instead of muttering about your circumstances or complaining, just mutter His word out loud just like you would mutter about the lousy weather or your terrible baseball team or the economy that's in a tailspin. Mutter, "The Lord is my Shepherd, I shall not want. He makes me lie down in green pastures. He restores my soul." (From Psalms 23). Mutter from the new covenant "God shall supply all my needs according to His riches in glory in Christ Jesus." (From Philippians 4:19). Speak His blessings over you out loud. You see, God knows our frame is to mutter about our circumstances. He encouraged Joshua to mutter His word instead. His words are words of life to you. They are spirit to you. Mutter the word. Why do this? As Joshua 1:8 above says so that you can have good success. Not just success - anyone can have success with the right circumstances. God wants you to have good success - without pain, without sorrows, without regret, and especially without stress. Mumble the word of God aloud. It's good for you. Call it as God sees it - even if you can't see it that way yet.

> Romans 4:17b (NKJV) says "...God, who gives life to the dead and calls those things which do not exist as though they did."

When the thought came that I had cancer, I would speak out aloud "I call cancer dead in my body. It has no right to live in my body. My savior Jesus paid the price on the cross so I could live cancer-free. I call cancer dead and I command it to leave my body in the name of Jesus Christ." I didn't lie. I didn't say cancer didn't exist. I just took my right that Jesus purchased for me on the cross and made my tongue the tongue of a king and a priest. Proverbs 18:21 (NASB) says, "Death and life are in the power of the tongue, and those who love it will eat its fruit." Words have spiritual power. Use them wisely. And you'll eat the results of your words. It's your tongue. Declare His promises over you with your tongue. This approach gets you to focus on His faithfulness, not your faith. It gets you to focus on His provision, not your lack. It gets you to focus on His righteousness, not your self-righteousness nor your guilt. No one can mutter aloud the words for you. You speak it out. We read in the new covenant in 2 Corinthians 4:13 (NASB), "*But having the same spirit of faith, according to what is written, "I BELIEVED; THEREFORE I SPOKE." We also believe; therefore we also speak.*" Make your problem bow down to Jesus, our Messiah.

> In Philippians 2:10 (NASB) we read, "so that at the name of Jesus EVERY KNEE WILL BOW, of those who are in heaven and on earth and under the earth."

The new covenant is pivotal to all of mankind. Are you going to mumble old covenant judgment all of which fell on Jesus, my

Lord and Messiah, at the cross? Or are you going to speak aloud new covenant promises and blessings, all secured by Jesus Christ alone, none of which is made available to you because of your nice thoughts or your nice actions? Mumble the new covenant promises of God, *then* you will have good success! Let's look at one verse for a simple example of how to do this. I spoke this word every day over my life while in my hospital bed. In Philippians 4:19 (NASB) it says, *"And my God will supply all your needs according to His riches in glory in Christ Jesus."* This verse became the following for me, "and my God will supply all of Phil's needs according to His riches in glory in Christ Jesus." Put yourself in the verse. Be a king. Be a priest. Call it out with your mouth. Mumble your way to success! Put some variety in it. Emphasize a particular word. Below, I do this in **bold** as an example for you.

> And **my God** shall supply all of Phil's needs according to His riches in glory in Christ Jesus.

> Or, And my God shall supply all of Phil's need **according to His riches** in glory in Christ Jesus.

Use your brain to make God's promises real to you. Use your mouth, one of the weakest members of your body to show Christ as strong in your life. You don't have to do this in front of others. You're not comparing yourself to anyone else anyway. You don't need to prove to anyone who you are in Christ. Before God, there is no distinction between you and any other believer concerning God's promises. Be strong with your mouth. Start in your prayer closet, and then do it in your car, do it whenever you're prompted to. It's His word and your mouth. Use 'em!

Proclaim His Death - Not Yours!

Another thing my wife and I did was to ask the nurses for grape juice and crackers. No, it was not a healthy diet or a food supplement we were doing. What exactly did we do with grape juice and crackers? We remembered what Jesus Christ did when He died on the cross. Have you ever asked yourself this simple question about the last three words He uttered before He gave up His life? Why did He say, "*It is finished!*"? Why those words? What was finished? Was it His life that was finished? That's what I used to think. Why even bother to say this if it's the last words you'll say? Most of us will say the most important things we can think of when we know it's our last words. We might tell our spouse we love her or our children we love them. What was going on here? What was finished?

God found the Lamb, Christ, acceptable and raised Him from the dead. He does not look at us to pronounce us clean, He looks at the Lamb of God, Jesus Christ. Everything good that Christ is, is put to my account. I am clean. I am shame-free. I am healed. I am whole. It's once, for all time. Christ does not need to die again.

My wife and I would take the grape juice and the crackers and "have Holy Communion." What does that mean? Let me show you by looking at the verses in 1 Corinthians to help you understand this more. In 1 Corinthians 11:23-26 (NKJV: New King James Version) my wife and I would read,

> [23] *For I received from the Lord that which I also delivered to you: that the Lord Jesus on the same night in which He was betrayed took bread;* [24] *and when He had given thanks, He broke it and said, "Take, eat; this is My body which is broken for you; do this in remembrance of Me."* [25] *In the same manner He also took the cup after supper, saying, "This cup is the new covenant in My blood. This do, as often as you drink it, in remembrance of Me."* [26] *For*

as often as you eat this bread and drink this cup, you proclaim the Lord's death till He comes.

That's a lot of verses here so be patient with me while we go through this. It's important to your life and your healing. When Jesus had given thanks and said *"take, eat; this is my body which is broken for you"*, two things are going on. Some religions make the bread that was broken out to be something sacred. Here's what is sacred - *Jesus, the Messiah.* He's the bread of life. Jesus held up the bread, broke it, then He pointed to His physical body and said - *"this is my body* [pointing to Himself, not to the piece of bread in His hand] which *is broken for you."* Did the apostles understand? I don't know. Perhaps not then. But they probably knew the next day because they saw Jesus pierced for our transgressions. They saw our Messiah crushed for our iniquities. He was pointing to His physical body when He said, *"This is My body, which is for you"* and he lifted the broken bread in His hands when He said, *"do this in remembrance of Me."* We are to break bread and eat it to remember what He did at the cross, all of it, a one-time for all-time action that resulted in our righteousness, our healing, our prosperity, our peace!

When you eat the bread, you crush it in your mouth. This helps you remember what He went through. Then we read, *"In the same way"* saying *"This cup is the new covenant in My blood."* As with the bread, we remembered His body which was broken for us, so with the cup, let's remember the blood which was shed for us. Just like in the first Passover, the shed blood of that lamb brought protection. The shed blood of the Lamb of God is for our righteousness before God. Our sins future, present, and past were washed clean by His blood. It's a continuous action. That blood was sprinkled on the doorpost in the first Passover. Jesus said He is the door of the sheep. Our relationship with God is now based on the shed blood of Jesus Christ, the Messiah. Instead of contemplating that you might die, praise God for the death of His Son. I don't want to make light of anyone's illness. It breaks God's heart to have you go through what you may be going through. But His Son's body was broken for you. Let's focus on the value of *His brokenness* on that cross.

Every time you partake, every time you break bread and drink the cup, you are saying His complete work is enough for you to live righteously with God, for you to live whole in His presence, for you to be able to always rest in His peace. He is not at war with you or angry with you. He loves you and gave His Son to you, for you, and to prove His love for you. You are victorious because of this finished work of Jesus Christ. You are not victorious in anything having to do with you, with your goodness, or with what you could do for Him. Your enemy has been defeated, not by your perfect life, but by His perfect life.

> The Complete Jewish Bible translation (CJB) of 1 Corinthians 11:26 reads as follows, *For as **often** as you eat this bread and drink the cup, you proclaim the death of the Lord, until he comes.*

Take Holy Communion often. My wife and I had Holy Communion almost every day. Remembering what He did on the cross gets your focus on Him and what He did and gets your focus away from yourself or what you can do. In the early church, they did this all the time. Acts 2:46 (NASB) says *"Day by day continuing with one mind in the temple, **and breaking bread from house to house,** they were taking their meals together with gladness and sincerity of heart. "*[11] Breaking bread and shouting, "here, here" when they lifted their cups. They remembered and they cheered God with gladness! The more you focus on what Jesus did, the more you trust God to bless you and to heal you. If you're going to take man's medicine, take the medicine God provided for you too. That's the

---

[11] **Bold** - my emphasis.

Holy Communion. You died with Christ and you were raised with Christ and now you are seated in the heavenlies with Him looking down on your situation. ***Proclaim His death, not yours.*** See it from God's perspective. Don't "shadow" box. Get in the ring of life and proclaim that God delivered you at the cross. Get real. God is completely satisfied with you because of what Jesus Christ did for you. God is not satisfied with you because of what you do or did.

Religion is focused on producing good citizens; in other words, people who are nice on the outside. Religion gets people to look at themselves and you naturally compare yourself to others when you do this. Instead, you should look at Jesus Christ and what He did. Don't look at yourself. It's a waste of your precious time and, honestly, a waste of God's time. Your niceness is not going to qualify you for anything with God. Neither will your sin disqualify you from receiving anything from God. Remember, Jesus, not you, satisfied God's righteous judgment against you at the cross.

Religion, however, stumbles and focuses on the verses which follow: 1 Corinthians 11:27-31 (NASB) says, *[27] Therefore whoever eats the bread or drinks the cup of the Lord in an unworthy manner, shall be guilty of the body and the blood of the Lord. [28] But a man must examine himself, and in so doing he is to eat of the bread and drink of the cup. [29] For he who eats and drinks, eats and drinks judgment to himself if he does not judge the body rightly. [30] For this reason many among you are weak and sick, and a number sleep. [31] But if we judged ourselves rightly, we would not be judged.*

The bottom line is this: what is an unworthy manner? Let's look earlier in that same chapter for some context to help us understand this from God's perspective. 1 Corinthians 11:18-20 (NASB) reads *[18] For, in the first place, when you come together as a church, I hear that divisions exist among you; and in part I believe it. [19] For there must also be factions among you, **so that those who are approved may become evident among you**. [20] Therefore when you meet, it is not to eat the Lord's Supper.*

What were they doing? Comparing themselves amongst themselves. This is the hallmark of religious people: "Hey look at me." "Look at how good I am." Look at my piousness or holiness as evidenced by what I "do." Imitate me is their familiar motto! This takes your eyes off the prize, Jesus, and what Jesus Christ accomplished for you. This is what religion does. Religion gets your eyes off Jesus and on yourself and how good you are or how good you can be. You end up comparing yourself with others. It's all so that some can be approved amongst you. Religious people are literally dying for your approval. It's all so carnal and stupid. The focus should always be on Jesus Christ, not on you and how good you are, or how nice you are, or how much *you* love God.

12.

HIS PURPOSE IN HIS LIFE FOR YOU[12]

Jesus wants us to use Him. This may be a hard thing for some people to hear, especially for the religious. After all, they've been taught for so long that they are an instrument of God and they are here to accomplish His purposes. Basically, you're a tool in God's toolbox to get His stuff done. That's not a real relationship. I don't have a relationship with the hammers and saws in my toolshed. Instead, Jesus showed us that God wants to be our supply for everything! Jesus said He was the door. In John 10:7-9 (ESV) we read, "7 So Jesus again said to them, "Truly, truly, I say to you, I am the door of the sheep. 8 All who came before me are thieves and robbers, but the sheep did not listen to them. 9 I am the door. If anyone enters by me, he will be saved and will go in and out and find pasture." He said that everything would come through Him. And we would go in and out and find green pasture, *through Him*. Again, when people get you to look at yourself by focusing on trying to be good for God or good enough for God to "use" them, you have taken your eyes off the prize. God doesn't "use" people.

---

[12] Romans 8:28 (NKJV) [28]And we know that all things work together for good to those who love God, to those who are the called according to *His* purpose.

Don't focus on you and how you are to be "used" by God. You have taken your eyes off the love of Jesus FOR YOU.

You discipline your mind to focus on Jesus, as your Shepherd, in the now. He is the one who makes you lie down in green pastures now, He is the one who leads you beside quiet waters now, He is the one who restores your soul now, and He is the one who guides you in the path of righteousness, not for your sake, but for His name's sake now. His good name depends on providing for you! It's His effort, not yours, that gives you success. Your success is not the result of your hard work or your effort. Your healing is not the result of your hard thoughts or efforts. God is the one who provides the increase in life. And He delights to give to you. This was what Jesus showed us when He was on the earth. Not only does God delight to give you your healing, your peace, your provision, your supply for every need, but He also calls you a co-worker with Him. You are not a tool in God's tool shed as a man would "use" tools. 1 Corinthians 3:9 (NIV) says, *For we are God's fellow workers; you are God's field, God's building.*

You see, we are **never** "used" by God. That is a traditional term used by well-meaning religious folks who are simply wrong. They gaze at the world's way of doing things, where men and women do use other men and women to get things done, and they assume God does the same thing. After all, God must be like me, right? No, instead, we are God's fellow workers or God's co-workers. We cooperate with Him. We are never used by God. He doesn't need us to get His work done. However, *He loves to work with us.* We are working together with God in this life.

There's another reason why religious people talk so much about God "using people." They don't know why some people are sick and suffering and they don't know why they aren't healed. Some people, naturally, must always have an explanation for why things happen. God never, ever desires that you be sick or that you die. Does it happen? Sure, it does. It's not His fault though. It's not always heaven on this earth, so let's not blame God because we don't understand what's going on and we have this need to explain away circumstances. Your life is more important to God than some explanation that just isn't true.

In 1 Corinthians 3:10-11 (CJB) we read, [10]*Using the grace God gave me, I laid a foundation, like a skilled master-builder; and another man is building on it. But let each one be careful how he builds.* [11]*For no one can lay any foundation other than the one already laid, which is Yeshua the Messiah.* Note the words "using the grace God gave me." It doesn't say using the law. It doesn't say using the people God gave me. It says I'm using the grace God gave me. Jesus, the Messiah, is the grace and truth we use. We use Jesus. That's hard for religious people to hear. But He is the grace God gave me and I use Jesus Christ. It's He that I build my life on. This is the only foundation I can lay. If you draw from His inexhaustible supply, you will be changed to be more like Him. And because He has an inexhaustible supply, you can take from Him all that you need.

Another thing the religious among us like to talk about is our purpose or our destiny in this life. There is no ultimate purpose or destiny for each life that is measured in the realm of the flesh. There is no grand scheme where you are going to discover the cure to cancer or lead an army of ten thousand or be a captain of industry. This is the way that a fleshy man thinks. Stinkin' thinkin' or thinking "in the flesh" can lead you astray. Your purpose in life is not in any of these man-made constructs. Instead, your only purpose is to receive and draw from Him, from Jesus the Messiah. To draw in His love, to draw upon His grace, to bask in His peace for you, to take your healing from Him. It's all for you! That's what He meant all along. Use Jesus.

John 4:31-34 (NASB) [31]*Meanwhile the disciples were urging Him, saying, "Rabbi, eat." * [32]*But He said to them, "I have food to eat that you do not know about." * [33]*So the* *disciples were saying to one another, "No one brought Him anything to eat, did he?" ³⁴Jesus said to them, "My food is to do the will of Him who sent Me and to accomplish His work."*

Jesus, our Messiah, is sustained, or fed, by doing God's will, by accomplishing God's work. *He* is refreshed when *He* does this. When Jesus was on the earth, He healed everyone who came to Him for healing. No one was left out. This was God's will. It is still God's will for our lives. Jesus is the same yesterday, today, and forever. He is energized when He gives you healing, when He gives you peace, when He gives you His love. He wants to do this. In Matthew 20:28 (NASB) it says, *just as the Son of Man did not come to be served, but to serve, and to give His life a ransom for many.* The word "and" means what's before and what's after are equally important. He came to serve *AND* to give his life a ransom for many. Not just the latter but the former as well. He came to serve. He still does. He hasn't changed.

Use Jesus and don't let yourself be used by man, no matter how nice you think they are. Men and women are prideful, and they like to point to what they've built up, what they've accomplished, what is attributable to their efforts. They're just glorifying themselves when they say that God uses them. We have nothing to give to God. Draw from Him and no one else. Take from your Messiah!

I freely received my healing from Jesus Christ. Freely. There were no strings attached. I don't owe God a dime. I know, in my heart, that without Him, I would not be healed, and I owe Him my life in one perspective. But I don't owe Him anything - my healing wasn't based on an exchange of some good I do for Him or others. Matthew 10:8 (NASB) says, *"Heal the sick, raise the dead, cleanse the lepers, cast out demons. **Freely** you received, freely give."*¹³ You have **everything** in Christ. In 1 Corinthians 3:21 (NASB) we

¹³ **Bold** - my emphasis.

read, "*So then let no one boast in men.* **For all things belong to you**." What belongs to you? All the good that God has for you is guaranteed by Jesus Christ because of His finished, completed work on the cross. He paid for it. Draw from Jesus, your supply!

I didn't see my healing evidenced in the emergency room when anointed oil was dripping all over my head. I didn't see my healing evidenced in my first week in the hospital while in Intensive Care. I didn't see my healing the second week, the third week, the fourth week, and so on through the first of four possible seven-week cycles of chemo. Just walk one step at a time. Continue to walk with "no condemnation" even if you haven't seen your healing just yet.

Take That Next Step Without Anxiety, Without Stress.

I did not take any pictures of myself in the hospital, nor did I allow anyone else to, except perhaps once. This was about six weeks into the first cycle of chemo when I was beginning to regain my strength. It is better to look at Jesus Christ. Because if you look at yourself, and especially if you looked like I did, you look terrible in the flesh. Here were the only two pictures I took of myself while I was going through that first cycle of chemo. Again, these were at about the sixth week and so I'm beginning to look better and have more strength. I had gone into the hospital on June 6th, 2014. The one photo on the left was taken on July 17, 2014. The one on the right was taken on July 14, 2014. My last day of chemo was July 28th. The third photo is a recent picture of me, taken October 28, 2017. It's unbelievable the difference! God is good!

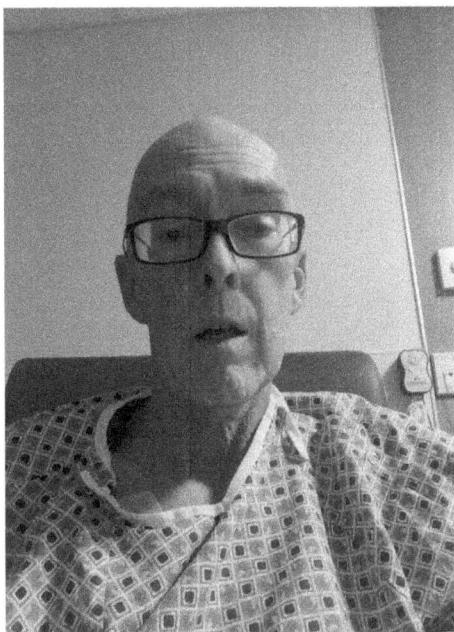

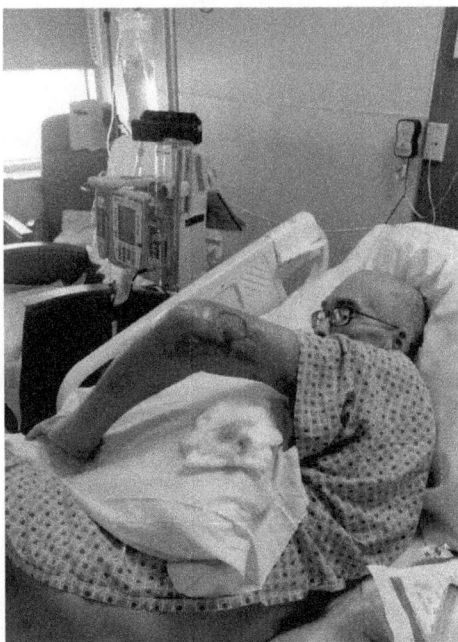

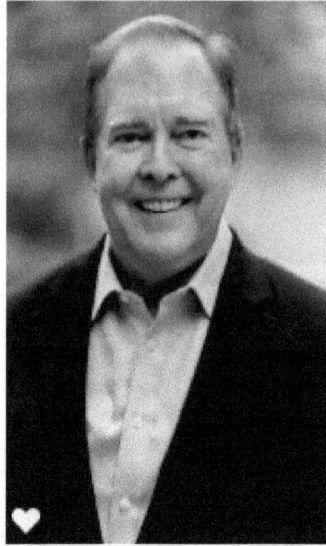

Give no thought to what's behind you and give no thought to what's in front of you. Go forward! As you stand, going forward, the Lord fights for you! Look, Israel was afraid when they came to the Red Sea, but they still prevailed. You may be scared. That's ok. In that first week, I had real palpable fear that I would not live. I suppressed that fear and didn't give it a voice or speak it out loud, but I was still afraid. A fear you can sense in your gut - like a punch in the stomach. Israel didn't know or understand how they would be delivered, but they were delivered. When you are still, as in standing still, you can receive more than when you are tied up in knots of doubt, worry and fear. When you hold onto doubt, worry and fear there is no room in your arms and hands to receive the abundance that God has for you. Empty yourself of doubt, worry and fear by keeping your eyes on your Savior, Jesus the Messiah. Give Him your anxieties, your cares, your concerns. He cares for you! Let Him fill you up with all that you need. Remember, He said He was the "I am." He is what we need Him to be for us. By doing this you will be *using* Jesus and not the other way around. He wants this. It sustains Him. *It is His purpose in His life for you.*

Look at Ephesians 4:7 (NKJV), *But to each one of us, grace was given according to the measure of Christ's gift.* Now God gave the measure. When God gives, is He cheap? Is God a miser in His measuring? Is He stingy with anything that He gives? NO! God gives abundantly. He gives more than enough. He gave us the Messiah, the Christ. How big is that? As big as you need it to be! It's God's measure. You were not given a stingy piece of grace. Take all of it. Take it now. Take it again tomorrow. Take it like God gave it. BIG. ABUNDANT. AND OVERFLOWING. That's our God and that's His gift, Jesus Christ.

Yeah, but doesn't God get tired of doing this for us? I mean, c'mon. Most of us are ungrateful, unworthy human beings, right? Yes, we're all ungrateful, more than we should be, but He never tires of giving to us. Because it's His nature to love you, it's His nature to give you your healing, to give you His peace, to give you your need for provision. He knew people couldn't think this way, so He told them in the gospel of Luke in verse 12:32 (NKJV), *"Do not fear, little flock, for it is your Father's good pleasure to give you the kingdom."*

I kept two verses of scripture in front of me when I was in the hospital. One was Philippians 4:13 (KJV) which says, *I can do all things through Christ which strengtheneth me.* See Christ doing all things for you. See Christ strengthening you. Give Him the assignment or project to strengthen your marriage, to heal your body, to provide for your business. Christ is your strength, and He is your Shepherd and provider. *There is no stress in His rest, only His strength.* Sickness and death are evil. It doesn't mean you are evil if you are sick or even if you have passed on. Sometimes bad stuff happens. Remember, *"there is NOW, therefore, no condemnation in Christ"* (Romans 8:1). Don't condemn yourself. But don't be afraid to speak out God's word over your life either. John 14:12-15

(NASB) says, [12] *"Truly, truly, I say to you, he who believes in Me, the works that I do, he will do also; and greater works than these he will do; because I go to the Father.* [13] *"Whatever you ask in My name, that will I do, so that the Father may be glorified in the Son.* [14] *"If you ask Me anything in My name, I will do it.* [15] *"If you love Me, you will keep My commandments.*

I can't explain why bad things sometimes happen. I don't care to try and explain it. I don't know how electricity works. I don't know how the combustion engine works. I don't need to know everything. I didn't care to "understand" the disease I had or what the blood levels, or what the white blood cell counts meant, etc. I know who does know everything and that's my focus. And I know whom I trust, whom I believe. I love God and one of his commandments was to do greater works than He did while on the earth. Why? Because Christ would go to His Father. Ask Him anything in His name. If you love Him, you will keep this commandment. Go ahead. Ask Him in the name of Jesus Christ and He will do it. You can ask Him because you believe in Him. Don't look at your circumstances. Just steel your mind to this Word of God that is true. You can ask Him because you are forgiven of everything and He doesn't remember your sins anymore.

How do you respond to evil? The same way Jesus did. By saying out loud what the word of God says. If your flesh is giving you pain, remind yourself that God says by His stripes you were healed. If your flesh has a need bigger than you, remind yourself that God shall supply all your need according to His riches in glory in Christ Jesus[14]. In Matthew 4:4 Jesus was reminding them that they needed more than physical bread. They needed Jesus, the bread of life. Matthew 4:4 (NASB) says, *But He answered and said, "It is written, 'MAN SHALL NOT LIVE ON BREAD ALONE, BUT ON EVERY WORD THAT PROCEEDS OUT OF THE MOUTH*

---

[14] Philippians 4:19 (NASB) And my God will supply all your needs according to His riches in glory in Christ Jesus.

OF GOD. "¹⁵ How do you respond to circumstances? How do you respond to cancer? With words that have proceeded out of the mouth of God. With *"It is written…"* When you speak out loud the word of God you are eating living bread. Yes, speaking His word is eating Jesus. You are holding the physical world accountable to the spiritual truth with your declaration of *"it is written."* You need to eat every day. So, what's in your mouth? I don't know how or when I received the evidence of my healing. The manifestation of my healing didn't seem dramatic, but it did happen. Whatever it is you have, be it a pimple or a tumor, speak to it. Command it to go. Call it dead and call your body alive in Christ. The problem is not going to uproot itself; instead, God's Word spoken out loud with faith unto Jesus will uproot it and plant it in the sea! What you speak to will obey you.

In 2 Corinthians 3:18 (NASB) we read, *"But we all, with unveiled face, beholding as in a mirror the glory of the Lord, are being transformed into the same image from glory to glory, just as from the Lord, the Spirit."*

Keep your eyes on Jesus and you'll be transformed by Him, not transformed by your efforts, but by Him. Just keep looking at Him and when your circumstances distract you with pain or other things, speak His word out loud over your body, over your situation, and before you know it, you'll be transformed and be more like Christ. Remember, you don't need to speak it out loud so your neighbor hears. You are not trying to impress others. You are the one who needs to hear it. Hearing yourself speak the word does something inside you.

If you have been speaking to your problem and have yet to see results, don't be discouraged. Discouragement can come when

---

¹⁵ Remember, the ALL CAPS is not God shouting at us. The translators sometimes do this to show that this verse came from the Old Testament.

you think it's up to you to get things done. It's easy to get discouraged when you are depending on yourself. Remember, there is NO condemnation in Christ. You don't need to understand how something works. You just need to keep speaking to it every day, commanding it to be uprooted. When Jesus taught His disciples to "say" to the mulberry tree (Luke 17:6), the Greek word used here for "say" is *lego*. Think of it as laying building blocks, sort of like Lego blocks, each time you speak and hold forth God's word with your mouth. It carries a sense of systematically laying forth or building upon. In other words, Jesus was telling them to repeatedly command the problem to depart. Don't just say it once and forget about it. Command with authority again and again until you get your breakthrough because of Jesus Christ! You are His king, so command like you have the heart of a king. You don't have to yell at it. Just speak to it as a king would. A king expects his word to be carried out, by others, and not by the king himself.

As I got closer to the end of my first cycle of chemo, I didn't know what to do. I had no energy to do much of anything. My gait was slow and deliberate. Physical therapists would come by every so often and focus on the little things, squeezing a sponge to gain strength in my hands, lifting my leg slowly and bending it, and other light exercises. I would walk the hallways once a day to gain strength. I had little strength, but at this point, I was getting comfortable doing nothing.

I was also getting comfortable with the "state" of my illness. As an example, I didn't eat much but I loved oatmeal and I enjoyed having a banana cut up with milk in my oatmeal. One time, my oatmeal arrived without a banana. Feeling like I was in a hotel room, I picked up the hospital bedroom phone and called down for bananas for my oatmeal. Dutifully they brought them up some thirty minutes later. I'm just too comfortable here, I thought. It was like I was in a hotel room getting hotel room service. That would soon change. I was cleared to go home after six weeks to rest for one week before being brought back for my final week of that first cycle of my chemo regimen.

During my initial stay at the hospital, I developed a bed sore on my elbow. I'm right-handed and grab food and everything with my right hand. I was propped up with pillows for the most part and leaning in on my left elbow. It took the hospital weeks before they discovered it. I ended up with a fungal infection in my left hand and an open wound at my left elbow. Between the hand and elbow, I would have a total of six surgeries over the next several weeks.

I was supposed to go back to the hospital for a final round of chemo after spending a week at home. Then I was supposed to go back home for two weeks of rest before the second "cycle" of chemo would begin. It was during this time at home that my daughter called me to share a dream she'd had that I should not continue with chemo. I listened patiently, but when people talk to me about the dreams they've had, I sort of tune them out. I'm not much into the interpretation of dreams. I prefer to deal with the real world and not with visions that may dance in people's heads. However, Alyson used a different argument that pricked my core. "Dad, didn't you tell us when we were younger that "*by Jesus Christ stripes you were healed*"? Why, then, are you going through chemo?", she said. It was Alyson's gentle, indirect way of saying, 'don't you believe that?' It's almost like saying to me - do you believe this word of God? Like her Mom, she was practiced in the art of the indirect. I did believe the word, but I had no actions behind this "thought" of belief. I didn't know what else to do but to tell my daughter that she was right. I committed to her that I would tell Dr. Robert the next time I saw him that I would no longer do chemo.

> John 6:28-35 (NASB) [28] *Therefore they said to Him, "What shall we do, so that we may work the works of God?"* [29] *Jesus answered and said to them, "**This is the work of God, that you believe in Him** whom He has*

sent." ³⁰*So they said to Him, "What then do you do for a sign, so that we may see, and believe You? What work do you perform?* ³¹*"Our fathers ate the manna in the wilderness; as it is written, 'HE GAVE THEM BREAD OUT OF HEAVEN TO EAT.'"* ³²*Jesus then said to them, "Truly, truly, I say to you, it is not Moses who has given you the bread out of heaven, but it is My Father who gives you the true bread out of heaven.* ³³*"For the bread of God is that which comes down out of heaven and gives life to the world."* ³⁴*Then they said to Him, "Lord, always give us this bread."* ³⁵*Jesus said to them, "**I am the bread of life**; he who comes to Me will not hunger, and **he who believes in Me** will never thirst.*¹⁶*

What are we to do to work the works of God? This was the question of those in the crowd who found Jesus. There are no complicated formulas here, no three steps to your release, or five steps to freedom, or whatever clever wisdom man comes up with. ***Only believe in Jesus Christ.*** That's it. Nothing more, nothing less. But what if you have stage-four cancer? It's the same - just believe in Jesus Christ. Believe that Jesus Christ did as God sent Him for. In Isaiah 53:4-5 (NASB) we read, ⁴*Surely our griefs He Himself bore, And our sorrows He carried; Yet we ourselves esteemed Him stricken, Smitten of God, and afflicted.* ⁵*But He was pierced through for our transgressions, He was crushed for our iniquities; The chastening for our well-being fell upon Him, And **by His scourging we are healed**.*¹⁷ Believe that He bore your grief, your pain. That's believing in Jesus Christ. Just trust God that He knew what He was doing when He sent His only begotten Son, the Messiah, for your healing.

¹⁶ **Bold** - my emphasis

¹⁷ **Bold** - my emphasis

13.

FAITH HEARS WHAT GOD SAYS

When I told Doctor Robert that I would not be going through any more chemotherapy treatments, he said this would not be his professional guidance for me. In fact, I think he was a bit stunned. He asked me to consider getting a second opinion before making this decision. He would set up an appointment for me to go to a friend of his at Moffitt Cancer Center in the Tampa area. I went to Moffitt, filled out the requisite forms, and waited to meet the doctor. It was the same story. It's like they colluded with each other beforehand. The doctor I met for a second opinion said I needed the chemo treatments. This was pressure on me to cave and go along with the recommended regimen. Perhaps they could lighten the regimen, but that decision would be made by my progress. But *"by Jesus Christ stripes I was healed."* He didn't understand this. Certainly, there was some compromise we could make, I asked. We agreed I would take another PET Scan to determine what was the current state of things. This would allow the doctors to see if a change in the regimen was warranted.

When you read the word, the gospels, and the church epistles, and when you speak the word, you are eating Jesus Christ, you are eating His words. Chew on this. Let this sink into your heart. His word brings you peace because you believe in Him. Eat His words and take from Him. Speak His word out loud so you can hear it. Listen to teachers of God's word who speak God's word about the finished work of Jesus Christ, the Messiah. Listen. Faith hears. It doesn't hear what you think, *it hears what God says.*

You have a new covenant with God. He is for you and not against you. His blessings are for the taking and they are guaranteed by His Son Jesus Christ. All we do is partake of it. David, in the Old Covenant, took his five small smooth stones, and though he heard the same taunts the others heard from Goliath; he spoke out loud his belief in God as His deliverer. Today, we have the one smooth Rock, our refuge, our strength, and our fortress, who gave His life for us that we might live in His favor which is freely given to us. David shouted at the Goliath before him that God would prevail. His focus was on what God would do, not how loud he spoke.

With God all things are possible. Faith hears. In Galatians 3:5 (NASB) we read, *So then, does He who provides you with the Spirit and works miracles among you, do it by the works of the Law, or by hearing with faith?* Take heed how you hear. Hear His word, believing it is true, and what you have, more will be given to you. Luke 8:18 (NKJV) says "*Therefore take heed how you hear. For whoever has, to him more will be given; and whoever does not have, even what he seems to have will be taken from him.*" Have ears to hear. Ask yourself, "what are you hearing?"

What must you do? Believe in the one who was sent for you! That's it. It's not complicated. Eat the bread of life. Drink living waters. The Father's will is that none given to Jesus would He lose. Faith comes by hearing. Hearing comes by the word of Christ. As you listen to His word spoken by yourself with your lips, spoken by believing ministers of God's word, you begin to develop a hearing ear, and, in effect, a hearing heart. And the voice you hear is God's word saying that He loves you, that He's faithful to His word, that

He is your healer, that you are forgiven. He's not going to forget you and He's not going to lose you. You are His forever! What do you do to be healed? Just believe or trust in Him who came. Trust that you were healed by His stripes. There is no greater thing to "do." Hear Him when you hear yourself speak His word.

On August 28th, 2014, one month to the day after I took my last chemo in that first of four cycles of chemo prescribed for me, I took my second PET Scan. I was relaxed. It wouldn't matter what they found. I was healed by the stripes of Jesus Christ. My faith was in Christ, not in my strength. I wasn't going to heal myself. He already did that 2000+ years ago. I would just walk one moment at a time trusting Him and His word to be true. My mind was fixed on the present. I didn't care about my past and I wasn't going to worry about tomorrow. To quiet my mind, I spoke God's word out loud over myself. Occasionally, my heart would pound with anxiety and I remembered Philippians 4:6-7. The Message translation reads, 6 *Don't fret or worry. Instead of worrying, pray. Let petitions and praises shape your worries into prayers, letting God know your concerns.* [7] *Before you know it, a sense of God's wholeness, everything coming together for good, will come and settle you down. It's wonderful what happens when Christ displaces worry at the center of your life.*

This isn't easy. We have a whole church epistle devoted to this. Galatians corrects errors that crept into the early church from straying away from the doctrine of Romans. Yes, error creeps into churches. Errors can creep into the opinions of well-meaning religious people. This is where you've got to be careful what you hear. If you are in doubt, just speak the written word out loud over yourself. Forget about what people say. Instead, declare this word, who is Jesus, as having preeminence in your life. The errors that crept into the church in Galatia were a reliance on works based on the Law. They were good works, but they were works that people held forth as more important than His singular, finished work, His once and for all time work of grace guaranteed on the cross. The bottom line is this: relying on works puts you under a curse. Instead, put yourself under Jesus, under grace.

On Wednesday, September 3rd at 9:30 a.m. Dr. Robert gave me the news. **They couldn't find any tumors at all!** He was puzzled. He didn't understand it and he didn't like not understanding things according to science. He now resorted to his training. It had to be there, he said. He just couldn't see it. He said it in a very unconvincing way. I could tell he didn't understand it. I told him it was gone. God healed me. Not denying nor acknowledging my confession of faith, he indicated I still needed to go through chemo, but they could find no tumors. None! I told him I would have no more chemo. I had been healed by the stripes of Jesus Christ. He was a good doctor. He was trained to believe that this was nothing more than a temporary blip. It was in remission he, sort of, mumbled, not out of commission as I thought. There was a very real possibility it could come back. I agreed to do another PET Scan three months later in November to placate this concern. Again, the results in November came back showing nothing! When we met in November, I told him I was going back to work in January. I needed to go through rehab because of my left elbow. It had "frozen" and I had lost all range of motion in my left arm. My arm was in a sling after recuperating from the many surgeries on the elbow and hand. I worked hard during those 2-3 months going to rehab 3 times a week, telling my therapist that God was my healer, and she would be amazed at the recovery.

It's amazing what happens to you when you speak the word out loud over yourself and you see God perform for you. You get bolder. It hasn't stopped. God has been so gracious to me. I'm not anywhere close to being a perfect guy or even a nice guy. But my qualification to receive from God is not by my faith or by my works, and not by anything having to do with me, only Jesus. I believe Jesus. He loves me. He is for me and never against me. He is always looking to bless me. Did I say that He loves me? Judge God faithful to His word. His faith requires *His* love for you, not your love for Him. His love for you energizes your faith in Him. When you are walking in 'now' faith, you are walking in His faith. Look at Him as the author (the writer) and the finisher (He completes it) of our faith. It's all about Him and not about us.

> In Galatians 5:6 (NASB) we read, *"For in Christ Jesus neither circumcision nor uncircumcision means anything, but faith working through love."*

Let's look at the context of this verse. Galatians 5:2-6 (NASB) says *"²Behold I, Paul, say to you that if you receive circumcision, Christ will be of no benefit to you. ³And I testify again to every man who receives circumcision, that he is under obligation to keep the whole Law. ⁴You have been severed from Christ, you who are seeking to be justified by law; you have fallen from grace. ⁵For we through the Spirit, by faith, are waiting for the hope of righteousness. ⁶For in Christ Jesus neither circumcision nor uncircumcision means anything, but faith working through love."*

Anything you do to "earn" the blessings of God means you've fallen from grace. You are under a curse. Don't "do" this. Put all the pressure on Jesus, not on you. That's what He wants. We wait on the hope of righteousness, Jesus Christ. This verse is talking about **His faith which is energized by His love for you**. When we receive this, it means everything. *Let His love for you drive you to trust in Him completely.* When you receive the gift of righteousness by calling Jesus Lord and by believing that God raised Him from the dead you are only obligated to live by trust or, in other words, by faith. I call it 'now' faith. Look at what Romans 1:17 (NASB) says, *For in it the righteousness of God is revealed from faith to faith; as it is written, "BUT THE RIGHTEOUS man SHALL LIVE BY FAITH."*

Don't even look at your faith. Sarah trusted God's faithfulness in the Old Testament. Hebrews 11:11 (NKJV) says, *By faith, Sarah herself also received strength to conceive seed, and she bore a child when she was past the age because she judged Him faithful who had promised.* Simply judge God faithful to what He promises in His word. Don't judge yourself negatively because of your misguided perception of how much faith you are supposed to have. Listen, hear, and receive from our loving Father, God.

How do you go on when you feel like you can't? Focus on His love for you. That will energize your mustard seed size faith. Take the measure of faith you've been given, however small you think it is, and direct it toward Jesus Christ. There were so many little moments of having to trust God in the now. During the times of physical therapy, they had me walk the hallway, then the next step was to go up a few stairs. I pushed myself to go to the top of the stairs that first time. I was scared but I was scared not to. God was my strength. Just put one foot in front of the other and go forward in His rest, I told myself. Just live in the now, trusting God in the now. Don't worry about tomorrow or yesterday's results. God told us this because it's easy to worry about tomorrow. Above all, don't judge yourself negatively. Walking is putting one foot in front of the other and catching yourself before you fall. Will you perfectly believe? I don't know. Again, don't focus on what "you" will do. Focus on His faithfulness to His promises and His love for you. His promises are true, and they are for you.

God is NOT judging you! He is loving you! In Romans 8:33, the apostle Paul poses that rhetorical question. *"Who's going to bring a charge against God's elect?"* Against us who are born again. And the answer: *"it is God who justifies."* God will work with you wherever you are at. If your faith requires you to touch His garment like the woman who had an issue with bleeding in the gospels, then so be it. If it requires that He visit your daughter as it was with the Rabbi Jairus in the gospels, then so be it. And if you have faith because you are someone with authority and you understand the authority of the spoken word as the Centurion in the gospels did, then God blesses that too.

You focus on Jesus who is grace and in that 'now' moment, He then sees your faith. This is a principle I learned from Pastor Joseph Prince. Jesus can see mustard size faith; He has good eyes! It doesn't matter what you think you see, especially if you think that you don't have faith. Focus on HIS Faith and HIS faithfulness, not yours. *It's not your business to determine if you have enough faith.* You spiritually died with Christ and now Christ spiritually lives in you.

> Galatians 2:20 says *"I have been crucified with Christ; it is no longer I who live, but Christ lives in me; and the life which I now live in the flesh **I live by faith in the Son of God**, who loved me and gave Himself up for me."*

We don't produce our own life. Christ lives in me and, thereby, works in me. Christ lives in me NOT because I act nice and NOT because I do good things. He lives in me by faith in Him right 'now'. Just believe in Jesus Christ, 'now'. Jesus is our Passover. He's what God sees, and He sees the blood Christ shed for us. Exodus 12:13 (NASB) says *"The blood shall be a sign for you on the houses where you live; and when I see the blood I will pass over you, and no plague will befall you to destroy you when I strike the land of Egypt."* God sees the blood of Jesus. In turn, you are to just see Jesus.

AB Simpson, who lived in the 19th century, wrote a small booklet entitled *Himself.* Here is a passage from what he wrote:

> *"There came a time when there was a little thing between me and Christ. I express it by a little conversation with a friend who said, "You were healed by faith." "Oh, no," I said, "I was healed by Christ." What is the difference?*

There is a great difference. There came a time when even faith seemed to come between me and Jesus. I thought I should have to work up the faith, so I labored to get the faith. At last, I thought I had it; that if I put my whole weight upon it, it would hold. When I thought I had got the faith, I said, "Heal me." I was trusting in myself, in my heart, in my faith. I was asking the Lord to do something for me because of something in me, not because of something in Him"[18]

Romans 3:26 (CJB) says *"and it vindicates his righteousness in the present age by showing that he is righteous himself and is also the one who makes people righteous on the ground of Yeshua's faithfulness."* The Complete Jewish Bible states it best: it has NOTHING to do with our faith but everything to do with His faithfulness! All other translations try to talk about our faith in Christ. It is His faithfulness. Our faith is nothing compared to the faith Christ has for His word. Jesus, or Yeshua, is Aleph and Tav. He is the first word and the final word in your life. Revelation 1:8 (NASB) says, *"I am the Alpha and the Omega,"* says the Lord God, *"who is and who was and who is to come, the Almighty."* He has the final say. When you speak God's promises over your life, you are giving God the final say.

Don't focus on your obedience either. You'll come up short and it will just get you into condemnation. Focus on His obedience, not your obedience. Many times, 2 Corinthians 10:5 (NKJV) is misquoted by well-meaning religious people who get you to focus on YOUR obedience. It reads, *"Casting down arguments and every high thing that exalts itself against the knowledge of God, bringing every thought into captivity to the obedience of Christ,"*

It's not our ability to obey Christ but it's His obedience even to death that He accomplished on the cross - this is what we focus

---

[18] *Himself* by AB Simpson. Pages 13-14. Copyright © 2013 by World Impact Ministries Printed in Canada. All rights reserved. ISBN 1-895-868-14-1

on. Focus on bringing every thought to His obedience, to "*the obedience of the Christ*" (what some translations rightly have), and what that means for you. What did the obedience of Christ yield or produce? Our righteousness! You need to be established in this righteousness, His righteousness. *Then* no weapon formed against you will prosper. (Isaiah 54:14,17)

Behind all the promises of the gospel is the promised Savior, who would die on the cross for our sins. If we attempt to base God's saving work on our performance, we are setting aside God's grace. We are inferring that His death for us was unnecessary or inadequate or incomplete. Don't set aside the grace of God for you.

14.

THE END OF MY BEGINNING.

This is the end of my beginning to walk with God and this is also the beginning for some of you. Make a simple decision. Do not look at yourself, only trust that God's word is true. My daughter, Alyson, came alongside me and encouraged me to walk on this promise of God's word. Sometimes we need others to speak the word of God into our life. I didn't know what to do except to take simple steps, one step at a time. Each step was oriented to trusting God. If you or someone you know is struggling with cancer or some terminal illness, come alongside them with an encouraging word from God's word. Speak words from the new covenant, specifically from the books of Romans through Thessalonians.

And if you are the one challenged with sickness or disease, then have someone who knows God pray for you. And when they pray, believe that your heavenly Daddy gives to you. In your weakness, use the weakest parts of your body, your eyes, your ears, and your mouth to reign in this life. Your eyes, ears, and mouth can't do anything on their own. They are powerless to accomplish things but use them rightly and you will reign in life because of Christ in you! Your eyes - only looking at Jesus as your supplier for every need; your ears - only hearing what He says with faith unto Him, your mouth – only meditating or confessing His word in your life so you will have good success.

In the end, I went back to work in January 2015, fully healed and with full range of motion in my left arm. God prospered me in my job. I decided to move on to another company where I became one of the top producers for that company. So much so, that in the timeline that I was there no one brought in more revenue in North America than I did. No one. Was it me? Nah. I stink at sales. I can't present well. I'm not that technical in the software world. I just trust that God will always provide for me. And I'm quick to speak His word OUT LOUD. Whether it's in my prayer closet, it's my "first response" to a problem, speaking the word. As Psalm 23:6 says, *"goodness and lovingkindness shall follow me all the days of my life."* Today, God is prospering me. I'm proving that as a man in my mid-60's I can compete with 30 and 40-somethings because He is my provider. I trust in Him. I don't owe God anything. But I know I owe God everything. This book is my attempt to encourage you, to come alongside you, and to say, God has this. He won't leave you. He won't forsake you. He's faithful to His word. Let's take this one step at a time.

I know I've been repetitive. And sometimes I sound like a cheer-leader. And I know life can be daunting. It has its challenges. I know of no life that is without challenges. Some challenges are tougher than others. Life on this earth isn't always easy. I have never been in a bed of roses. I just constantly, unendingly, remind myself that He is for me and not against me and give Him my problems one 'now' moment at a time. And my love for Jesus is to let Him love me. That's how I show Him my love. I let Him love me. I let Him bless me. He wants to. I talk to Him like He's my Daddy. In Romans 8:15 (NIV) we read, *"For you did not receive a spirit that makes you a slave again to fear, but you received the Spirit of sonship. And by him, we cry 'Abba, Father.'"* Abba is the Jewish term for Daddy or

Poppa. Our Spirit of sonship cries out to God, as our Daddy! He's my heavenly Daddy who delights to be in my presence. I don't deserve this life that I live. I just am not good enough to deserve it. But because I know this and because I believe Him, I receive all His blessings for me. I don't ever want to deserve these blessings. And neither should you. Just receive all His blessings. Take them from Jesus. *Take from Him all the time.*

Jesus made no one wait for their healing. All who came to Him were healed. Our western notion of waiting is for our own consumption. When I was sick, I could have received my healing at any time. It was not up to the Lord; it was up to me. I ended up at a point where I could do nothing to help myself. I had to trust God. I had reached the end of my rope and needed His rope to save me. The just or righteous shall walk by faith, not by waiting and waiting and waiting and waiting. God doesn't play games with our needs. He is not time-bound. That's why He can say *"By Jesus Christ's stripes you were healed!"* In almost all the occurrences in the New Testament the word waiting is in the context of to wait ON the Lord or to have your 'hope' in Him; again, not to wait FOR the Lord but to wait ON Him, to hope in Him. When we are waiting on Him, we are expecting from Him, we are receiving the supply of our need from Him right now. He is our deliverer. What is our only responsibility in the new covenant? Simply to walk by faith in Him at this 'now' moment. This is not only for healing but for every need we have in this life. The need for peace, the need for prosperity, the need to be anxious for nothing. When we trust Him, our faith is directed to Him. It is not dependent on our good works or our efforts. *We look to Jesus, our Savior, in everything.* He doesn't make us wait. Even though our experiences might say otherwise, the Good Shepherd doesn't make us wait. But most times our focus is not on Jesus but ourselves, our condition, our lack. Instead, God wants us to see His Son, our supply, and not to look at ourselves or our lack. We are not even to look at our faith. We need only to look to Him. Jesus is your *only* qualification to receive from God.

I don't know why I did this at the time, but I endeavored to only see Him. And when He looked at me, He wasn't mad at me, He wasn't frustrated with me. He always had this great smile and was happy, you could say joyful, to see me. When you look at Jesus, you need to think about what you are expecting from Him. At first, He was just there to love me and be with me. But after my youngest daughter Alyson spoke to me about having already been healed by Jesus Christ stripes, I now was expecting differently, and with more of a sense of urgency. God knew that I wasn't the type of person that would yank out the IV's stuck in me and run out of the hospital. He made a way for me to stop doing chemo.

I spent September to December of 2014 rehabbing my elbow which had frozen from all the surgeries. And I went back to work the first full week of January the following year. When I had my final PET scan in May 2015 and sat down with Dr. Robert to review the results, he simply remarked that it looked like I had never had cancer. He frankly said he'd have to agree that whatever I thought had happened did happen. We agreed to do annual visits in November and to have blood tests done. Each time I went back to see him in November, there was nothing wrong with my blood. Nothing. Counts are correct. I have no bad cholesterol levels. He doesn't get it and I don't care if he doesn't get it. I was healed by the stripes of Jesus Christ! In my last visit with him in November of 2018, he said I didn't have to see him anymore. I think he just felt these annual visits wouldn't produce anything but the great results he saw.

It took many months for me to gradually regain my weight. Rehab was hard work. When I first went home, I was so weak I couldn't climb the stairs to make it to our bedroom, so I slept in the living room on a twin bed. My youngest daughter, Alyson, and her future husband, Bret, graciously fixed the shower in the garage so

I could use that. I needed help from Penny to take a shower in the garage! I needed help to walk. Initially, I bought a cane. but I lost it and later realized I didn't need it. One time, I had to buy a new pair of shoes. I needed a special kind of shoe because my feet were still swollen. To do this I had to walk to the shoe store in the mall. I walked, and walked, and walked in that mall. It was exhausting. I don't think anyone understood or knew this. I knew. It was August in Florida and it was hot. Heavy breathing accompanied my gait. I regretted going out to buy those shoes because it took so much work and so much out of me.

One day at a time. One of those days, I decided to call my boss where I used to work. This was in mid-November. He said he would welcome me coming back after the first of the year. I would call him again around Christmas. I wouldn't let go of God who was my strength. I had just been healed by the stripes of Jesus Christ and I was determined to see Him work in my life one day at a time. It was exhilarating. Exhausting but exhilarating. When the Lord holds your hand, you won't fall and hurt yourself. You won't be hurled headlong. Because it's the Lord who holds your hand.

> Psalms 37:23-24 (NASB) says, "23 The steps of a man are established by the LORD, and He delights in his way. 24 When he falls, he will not be hurled headlong, because the LORD is the One who holds his hand."

My wife would help me walk around the cul-de-sac. Not up and down the street. Just the circle of the cul-de-sac where we lived. It was exhausting walking more than 200 feet. But come January 5th, I returned to work and I've been working ever since. Below is a picture of me walking in my early rehab efforts.

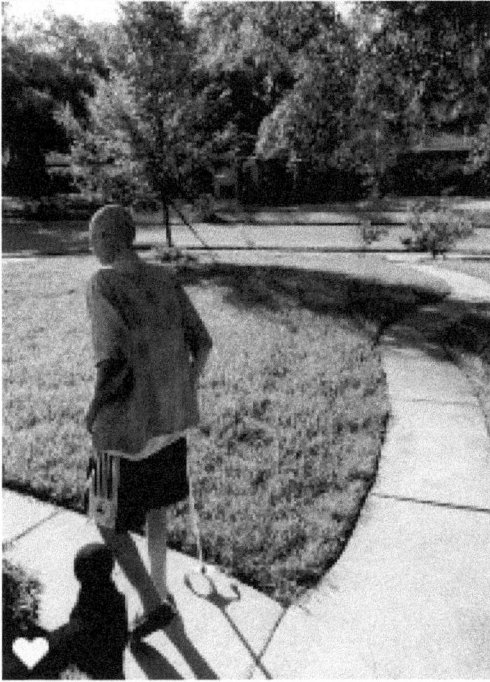

There is so much else that took place, but I wanted to lay the right foundation, Jesus Christ. He loves you. You see, my testimony isn't that I was healed of cancer, my testimony is the word of God, the Word made flesh, Jesus the Christ, my Savior, my lover, and my strength. He is the word of my testimony. It's not about me. It's all about Him. Because of Him, because of His love for me, I am more than a conqueror (Romans 8:37). It's a continual love. You draw from and take from Jesus what you need. He is there for you. Don't be anxious about tomorrow. Forget your past. Enjoy Him today. Stay in the 'now' of His love for you. There is no condemnation in this Messiah, the Christ.

I want you to look at Jesus always expecting to receive good from Him. The love of the Father is in Him *for you*. *You* are the object of *His* love. It is good for your heart to be established by grace, not by foods, not by prescriptions, not even by exercise (Hebrews 13:9). You may need to eat every day, but you need His grace for you always. Remember, *Jesus is grace and truth.* Your heart needs to be established by grace, by Jesus, and not by your works or your diet. Let Him work at His pace in your life. The first time Jesus came, the angels proclaimed to the shepherds in the field, "Don't be afraid." I'm not an angel by any stretch of the imagination but you don't need to be afraid. His purpose in your life is to save you. Let Him do that. His famous words in Matthew 11:28 still apply to you and me today.

> Matthew 11:28-30 (NASB) says, ²⁸"*Come to Me, all who are weary and heavy-laden, and I will give you rest.* ²⁹"*Take My yoke upon you and learn from Me, for I am gentle and humble in heart, and YOU WILL FIND REST FOR YOUR SOULS.* ³⁰"*For My yoke is easy and My burden is light.*"

He is gentle and humble in heart *for you.* His yoke *for you* is **easy** and His burden is **light** for you.

I don't know why I wasn't healed before I went into the hospital. I don't know why I didn't receive my healing after the first week in the hospital, or after the second week, or the third week. At first, I thought some of it depended on me, and as I got weaker and weaker, I realized that nothing could depend on me. Nothing. But the more I focused on how much He loved me, the more I overcame, not through my ability but through His love for me. In the Song of Solomon 4:7 (NASB) it says, "*You are altogether beautiful, my darling, and there is no blemish in you.*" This is how He made me in Christ, and this is how He sees me now. Altogether beautiful. God made this new covenant with His Son, Jesus the Christ, my Messiah. It only depends on these two parties, and not at all on me. Everything depends on Jesus the Christ, the Messiah, who represents me. Even in sin, He is my advocate with God. He is The Lord my Righteousness (1 John 2:1). Now go and enjoy the healing God has already given to you!